organic
beauty

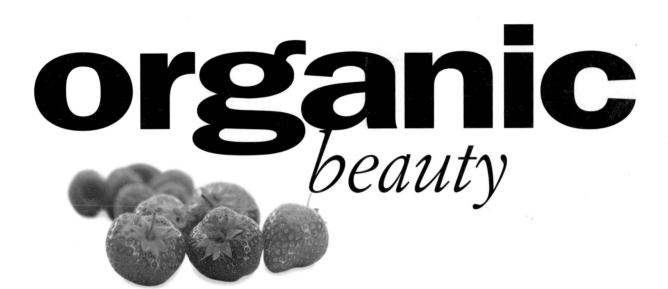

organic
beauty

Josephine Fairley

photography by John Davis

A DK Publishing Book

LONDON, NEW YORK, SYDNEY, DELHI, PARIS,
MUNICH AND JOHANNESBURG

Produced for Dorling Kindersley by Walton and Pringle
www.waltonandpringle.com

Managing Editor Gillian Roberts
Managing Art Editor Tracey Ward
Category Publisher Mary-Clare Jerram
Art Director Tracy Killick
DTP Designer Louise Waller
Senior Production Manager Maryann Webster

Photographer John Davis
Stylist Liz Hippisley
Models Jo Whitaker at M&P Management Plc
Caroline Barton at Storm

First American Edition, 2001
01 02 03 04 05 10 9 8 7 6 5 4 3 2

Published in the United States by
DK Publishing, Inc., 95 Madison Avenue, New York, New York 10016

A Cataloging-in-Publication record is available from the Library of Congress

ISBN 0-7894-7191-4

Color reproduced in Singapore by Colourscan
Printed and bound by Printer Trento, Italy

Printed on acid-free, chlorine-free, recyclable and biodegradable
paper from a sustainable forestry source.

See our complete
catalog at
www.dk.com

contents

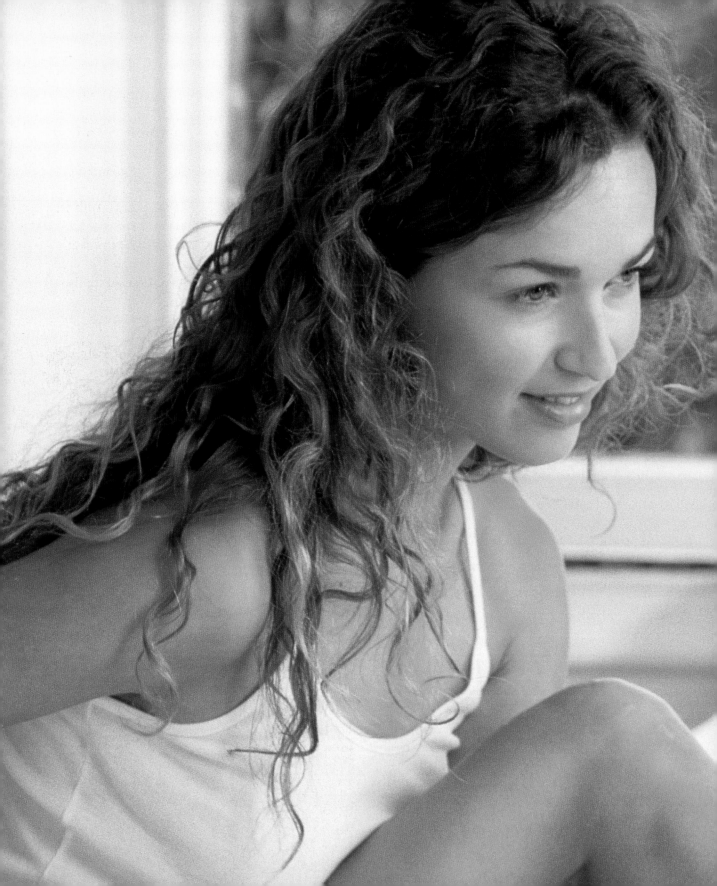

Why go organic?

If you are concerned about what foods you are putting into your body, you have probably started to think about what you put on it, too. Organic beauty is the logical next step after eating organically, especially when you consider that part of the skin and bodycare products we use are absorbed directly through the skin into the bloodstream. In addition to the personal benefits, it also makes sense to use sustainably produced products that will not impact on the planet's ecosystem.

benefits
in beauty terms

Nature has wonderful, skin-saving ingredients that can be harvested without impacting on the planet, and understanding these elements makes an organic approach to beauty simpler.

If you care about what you put in your body, you've probably started to care what you put on it, too. Organic beauty is the logical next step from eating organically, because when we put something on our skin, we're essentially "feeding" it, as it drinks in the ingredients in our moisturizers, makeup, bodycare, and shampoos.

Not so long ago, doctors used to tell us that the skin was a one-way street: it let sweat and toxins out and acted like an impermeable "raincoat," a barrier that didn't allow anything in – but that thinking has changed. Today, more and more drugs are delivered via the skin because it is a swift and easy way to access the bloodstream. Take, as examples, hormone replacement and nicotine patches. Today, it is acknowledged that aromatherapy's power to shift our mood or improve our wellbeing is not only because of the effect of those pretty smells on our psyche, but also because therapeutic quantities of the plant essences are absorbed through the skin into our systems. According to experts, like Rob McCaleb of the Herb Research Foundation, "up to 60 percent of what we put on our skin is absorbed into the bloodstream." Sebastian Parsons, Managing Director of organic skincare company Dr. Hauschka, says that the average woman absorbs over 30 lb (14 kg) of moisturizing ingredients into her bloodstream over 60 years – and that's excluding any other cosmetics. No one knows yet what the long-term effect of that cocktail of chemicals will be.

GREEN YOUR ROUTINE

If you avoid chemicals in your diet, it is logical to do the same for your beauty regime. If you are also concerned about our planet, it makes sense to seek cosmetics that are sustainably produced. Many mass-market cosmetics, for instance, contain Genetically Modified Organisms – usually derived from corn or soy. Others feature mineral oil and petrolatum, both of which come from nonrenewable sources. However, nature offers wonderful, skin-saving ingredients that can be harvested, year after year, without impacting on the planet's ecosystem.

There is, of course, one foolproof way to make sure that your skincare, haircare, and bodycare is entirely natural – make it yourself, using pure ingredients. What's more, you'll be able to incorporate more of the high-quality botanical ingredients than you'd normally find in readymade products (many of which are filled up with water) – and it will also save you money. The price you pay for cosmetics in the stores includes transportation, tax, packaging – and often a big chunk of advertising costs. So follow the simple, fun-to-try formulations in this book, and you'll soon discover how some of the world's greatest tried-and-tested beauty boosters can be found in your kitchen cabinets or your fruit and vegetable patch or herb garden.

OFF-THE-SHELF PRODUCTS

Being practical, though, there is not always time in our busy daily schedules to whip up cosmetics in the blender. So the good news is, just as the food industry has woken up to consumer demand for organic food, so, too, are entrepreneurial beauty companies creating lines with fewer preservatives and chemicals, but which are as effective.

Inevitably, though, some companies' natural and organic claims just don't stand up to scrutiny, and because so far, organic regulations to cover cosmetics are still being defined, it can be hard to tell what's really pure – and what isn't. This book is here to help and aims to steer you through the natural beauty maze, pointing you in the direction of the beauty companies whose products are really as pure as nature intended.

Being an organic beauty, however, is about much more than what you put on your skin. It means taking a holistic approach. It is about eating good food, sleeping well, and keeping your body moving. Exercise gives a boost not only to your skin, but also to your mood, your spirits, and the way your whole system functions.

This book not only helps you with finding the right organic beauty treatments, it also offers advice on subtle lifestyle changes to make you look and feel better than ever.

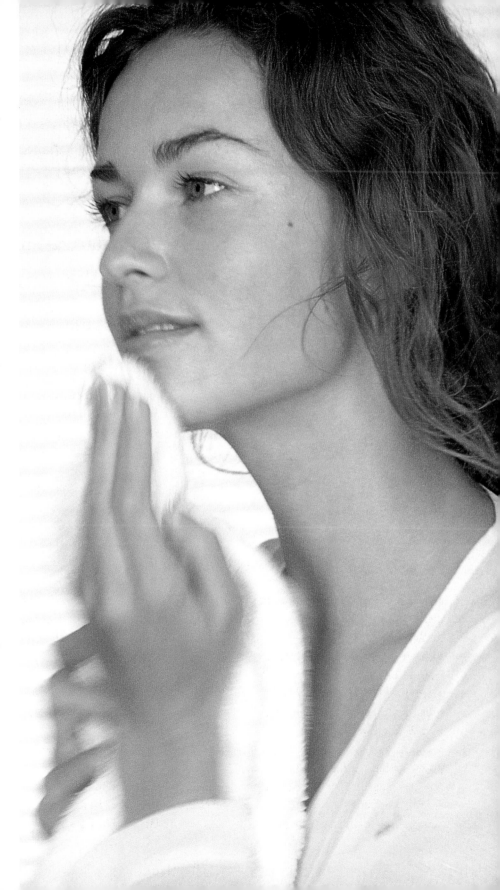

natural
health issues

Most cosmetics and skincare products contain preservatives to lengthen their shelf-life, but to avoid their potentially harmful effects, here's how to select products that are more natural.

Just as the long-term effect on our health of the chemicals present in our food has never been quantified, nor has the impact on our wellbeing of the dozens of different cosmetics that a typical woman applies to her skin each day. Without wishing to sound alarmist and send you dumping the contents of your bathroom cabinet straight into the trash can, it's worth being aware that there are question marks over the safety of certain individual ingredients present in beauty products – let alone the "cocktail" effect.

QUESTIONABLE INGREDIENTS

Some artificial colors – derived from coal tar and used in makeup and skincare products – have been shown to cause cancer not only when ingested, but when applied to the skin. Other ingredients are known irritants, and yet may still be found even in "hypoallergenic" and baby products that we buy because we think they're

safe and gentle. There is also concern over some of the common preservatives, described opposite.

We're faced with so many risks in life that many people may consider the health impact of a lipstick to be fairly low down on the lists of things to worry about. But for anyone wishing to cut down their overall exposure to chemicals for ecological reasons, or, for instance, in the case of cancer patients who are now increasingly being given "lifestyle" advice to avoid chemicals, (not to mention anyone who is or plans to become pregnant), "greening" what we put on our bodies, as well as in them, can become a priority. (A recent case that made headline news, for instance, found traces of 350 manmade chemicals – including personal care products – in human breast milk.)

But awareness is all. And so is the reading of ingredients lists, enabling you to make a more informed choice about what products you put in your makeup

bag and on your bathroom shelf. Now that cosmetics – certainly, those sold in Europe – have to list ingredients in Latin, even natural ingredients have complex Latin names, adding to the confusion about what is a natural and a chemical substance. This book aims to explain these ingredient lists and help you identify truly natural choices.

WHY ADD PRESERVATIVES?

If a cosmetic contains water, it needs preservatives to prevent spoilage. Without preservatives, creams, gels, and lotions become contaminated with bacteria. If a contaminated product seeps into the eyes, there's a chance that it could trigger a serious infection, as can bacteria entering a cut or scrape on the skin. The safety of cosmetics is more strictly controlled than food, with some cosmetics having a shelf life of up to seven years.

Many of the health anxieties relating to cosmetics concern preservatives.

Some of the most allergenic and skin-irritating ingredients release small quantities of formaldehyde – which is not only an irritant, but also a neurotoxin and a carcinogen. A few cosmetic maufacturers avoid these ingredients, but many do not. To identify potentially harmful ingredients in cosmetics and skincare products, refer to the information on page 16.

THE LONG-TERM EFFECTS

The paraben family of preservatives (which is not formaldehyde-based) has a lower potential for irritancy. As a result, parabens can be found in up to 99 percent of all cosmetics. Parabens are formulated into several compounds and are listed on cosmetic labels as either methyl-, ethyl-, propyl- or butylparaben. Although considered less harmful than formaldehyde-based preservatives, a recent report has questioned the safety of parabens. The concern is over parabens in cosmetics and skincare products absorbed through the skin of pregnant women. Research has shown that they may affect the future fertility of male babies. Professor John Sumpter of Brunel University, England – an expert on estrogenic chemicals in the environment – believes the results could be significant, because over the last few decades, paraben use has been very widespread in the cosmetic industry. These chemical preservatives might just play a role in falling sperm counts and rising breast cancer rates.

To avoid preservatives in cosmetics, the simplest solution is to make your own. If there's water in a recipe – which may breed bacteria and cause infection – remember to store the product in the refrigerator, and use it up quickly to avoid any risk of bacteria. Alternatively, look out for the more natural preservatives found in store-bought cosmetic products, which include ingredients such as grapefruit seed extract, phenoxyethanol, potassium sorbate, sorbic acid, tocopherol (vitamin E), vitamin A (retinol), vitamin C (ascorbic acid), gum benzoin, and pycnogenol (a potent antioxidant).

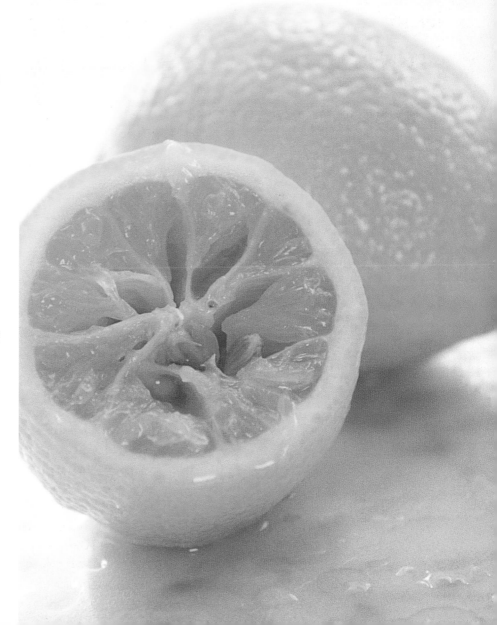

genuine
organic products

Scanning the shelves trying to figure out what's really organic can be very confusing. The following pages show you what ingredients to avoid and how to recognize them.

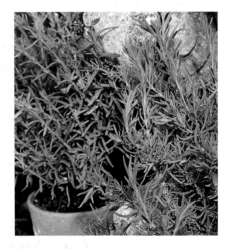

When you buy organic food, you can be reassured that it really is organic. On the packaging, you'll find organic certification: a recognizable symbol, and an ingredients list. You know that 95 percent of any product described as "organic" is and that within that last 5 percent, organic ingredients must be used, when available. But when you buy "organic" bodycare, it's hard to tell whether that's a genuine claim. Some products may use the word

"organic," yet contain only a tiny amount of organic herbs, topped up with preservatives and chemicals. So far, virtually no legal standards exist for cosmetics and toiletries, although certification bodies, such as The Soil Association in Britain, are in the process of writing them.

So how can you tell which products really are organic? Some companies are helpful enough to state the percentage of organic ingredients on the label. If they don't, study the ingredients list, where some manufacturers mark organic ingredients with a symbol. Ideally, you want to see organic ingredients listed near the beginning (those used in the greatest quantities) rather than at the end of the list. You should also be wary of the term "pesticide-free." It may denote organic ingredients, but it could also suggest the use of artificial fertilizers and, more worryingly, the phrase may be meaningless, because "pesticide-free" has no legal definition.

If you are in doubt about a product, write to the company and ask about the certification of ingredients claimed to be organic. Companies with nothing to hide should be responsive and helpful.

The advice in this book will help you figure out which "natural" cosmetics on the market really are what they claim to be and which are hyping their products as something they're not.

SOMETHING WILD?
The terms "wild," "wild-crafted," or "wild-harvested" are sometimes seen on labels, often referring to herbs. This means that they were picked in the wild, not cultivated in fields. Such ingredients cannot be organically certified because the same controls cannot be applied to natural areas as to fields. Wild ingredients may, possibly, have been exposed to pesticides or spray drift. They are, however, still botanical ingredients, not something created in a laboratory.

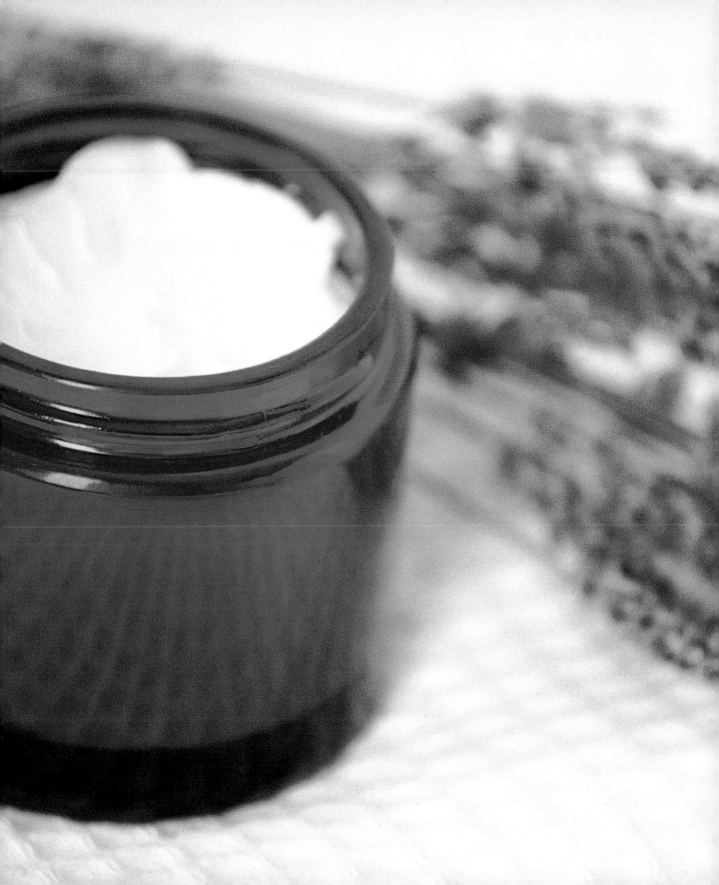

ingredients
to avoid

When it comes to natural cosmetics, exactly what should you look out for? GMOs, animal-testing, and excess packaging should all be avoided; the following pages explain how.

Latin. Many of us loathed it at school. Now we hate it on cosmetics labels, but any cosmetics sold in the European Union must, by law, list ingredients in Latin. Usefully, some put in the translations, too. In the United States, it's easier: botanical ingredients are listed by names that we understand, such as almond oil or grapeseed oil.

In the *glossary* on page 125 of this book, you'll find a comprehensive list of botanical ingredients and their Latin translations. For a list of the ingredients that a would-be organic beauty should probably avoid, in addition to those items you definitely don't want in your cosmetics, turn to page 16.

Don't take the word "natural" for granted on the front of a jar, a tube, or a bottle; flip it over and look at the ingredients list. What you're looking for is natural ingredients placed high on the ingredients list, rather than just tucked away at the end after a string of chemicals. Many products that claim to be "natural" are little more than a chemical composition with a hint of "natural" fragrance.

While you're getting to learn your way around labels, it may be useful to carry a photocopy of the *glossary* from the back of this book with you while you shop. As a rough guide, choose cosmetics and personal care products that contain the fewest ingredients. Most natural beauty companies like to keep their formulations as simple as possible, while still being effective.

DON'T THROW IT ALL AWAY
Packaging issues should also be on organic beauty-shoppers' minds. The advantage of homemade cosmetics is that you can collect and reuse attractive glass bottles and jars to store the face and body treats you've made yourself. When you buy cosmetics, always choose glass over plastic, where possible, then wash thoroughly and recycle. Although recycling facilities for all but the most common plastics (usually beverage bottles) are extremely rare, try to take advantage of them where you can. The most easily repackaged plastic has a number 1, or the letters PET, on the bottom. Naturally, you should also avoid products that are wastefully packaged or, at the very least, recycle the box, the carton, and even the little instruction leaflet. Alternatively, you could try sending the packaging back to the manufacturer, expressing your concern for their negative impact on the environment.

THE FURRY BUNNY FACTOR
Fact: cosmetics are still tested on animals. So are the ingredients that go into them. What complicates life further for the consumer is that the rules differ from country to country. In Britain, there's a complete ban both for finished products and ingredients:

no more mascara dripped into rabbits' eyes, no more rats shaved and swabbed with cream until their skin blisters, no more mice fed with antiaging creams to see how much they can consume before dying. But that ban applies only to cosmetics made in the Britain, not those that have been imported.

In the rest of Europe, it may be five to seven years before a full ban is implemented. Meanwhile, up to 35,000 animals will continue to die each year in European cosmetics tests.

In the U.S., although some products carry the international "Humane Cosmetics Standard" label initiated by the British Union of Anti-Vivisection (BUAV), awareness lags far behind that of Europe.

CONSUMER POWER

So what can the concerned shopper do? To start with, write to the BUAV for their Little Book of Cruelty Free (for the address, see *Directory* on pages 122-124), and buy your products from the "approved" companies listed inside. You can also check packaging for the cruelty-free logo or for the words "cruelty-free."

According to the BUAV, boycotting companies who continue to test on animals is useless unless you inform them why. So write to the companies you've decided not to buy from, and explain why. If you're still confused, contact BUAV, which has a huge library of information on most cosmetics and skincare companies.

JUST SAY NO TO GMO

All over the world, consumers are protesting about the introduction of Genetically Modified Organisms (crops that have had their genes scientifically altered) into the food chain. But did you realize that they're in cosmetics, too? Soy and corn, in particular, are common sources of makeup and skincare ingredients.

The outcry in Europe, particularly Britain, has brought GMOs onto cosmetics companies' agendas. Many have now made strides to eliminate GMOs from their products, running stringent testing of batches of ingredients to guarantee their purity.

European companies are far ahead of their American counterparts where GMOs are concerned. Many US companies simply state that, since there's no evidence of any harm to humans from the use of GMOs in cosmetics, we shouldn't be worried. For many of us, however, anxieties about GMOs are not solely personal, they're environmental.

Pierre Perrier, head of Christian Dior Laboratories Research and Development, suggests that concerned consumers should write to cosmetics companies and ask for their policies on GMOs, and switch to brands that satisfy their concerns.

Consumer power has forced food companies to go GMO-free, and that's the only way to get the beauty industry to follow suit.

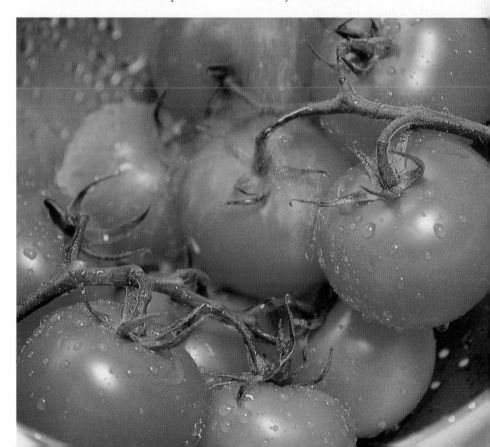

organic *packaging*

The complicated wording on packaging can be very confusing. The list outlined below helps you identify potentially harmful ingredients and explains why you may want to avoid them.

10 THINGS YOU DON'T WANT IN YOUR NATURAL COSMETICS

1 Artificial colors. Several colors are believed by some experts to be potential carcinogens. Steer clear in particular of FD&C Red No. 6 and FD&C Green No. 6. Avoid rainbow-colored products to minimize your exposure to artificial dyes.

2 DEA, MEA, and TEA (not the natural ingredient tea, but the capital-lettered chemical version). These can cause allergic reactions, irritate the eyes, and dry the hair and skin.

3 Formaldehyde. An expensive but effective preservative used in nail hardeners, nail polish, and many cosmetics. Skin reactions are fairly common, and some doctors worry about other, more serious long-term effects. The following are all formaldehyde-derived: Imidazolidinyl urea (the second most identified preservative causing contact dermatitis, according to the American Academy of Dermatology); diazolidinyl urea; 2-bromo-2-nitropropane-1; 3-diol; imidazolidinyl urea; DMDM hydantoin; and quaternium 15.

4 Fragrance. Synthetic fragrances used in cosmetics may have up to 200 ingredients; they don't have to be labeled separately, and many are petroleum-based. Some potential problems caused are dizziness, skin irritation, and hyperpigmentation. Be aware that the words "fragrance-free" do not necessarily help you avoid the problem: usually, smell-masking chemicals will have been added as well. Look instead for the words "natural fragrance," or choose products whose scent comes from essential oils.

5 Isopropyl alcohol. An antibacterial solvent, derived from petroleum.

6 Methyl paraben. One of the most widely used preservatives, it may trigger irritation on sensitive skins, as can butyl-, ethyl-, and propylparaben. There is also a suggestion that these may be xenestrogens – more research into this is due to be carried out.

7 Methylisothiazolinone. A preservative with a large potential for causing allergic reactions or irritation.

8 Paraffin. Used in cold creams, wax hair removers, eyebrow pencils, and many other products. Often derived from petroleum or coal.

9 Propylene glycol. Other than water, this is the most common moisture-carrying vehicle used in cosmetics. Although it can be derived from vegetable glycerin or seaweed, it is more usually a petroleum derivative.

10 Sodium lauryl sulfate. A detergent and emulsifier that may cause drying of the skin due to degreasing effects, and can be irritating. The drying action interferes with the skin's barrier function, making it easier for other chemicals to enter. When combined with a number of other ingredients, SLS can form carcinogenic nitrosamines (nitrogen compounds).

PETROCHEMICALS – AND WHY YOU SHOULD AVOID THEM

Petrol and paraffin are associated with industry, but did you realize that you're almost certainly putting them on your body? Mineral oil (*paraffinum liquidum*) and petrolatum feature high on ingredients lists of many skincare, bodycare, and haircare products. Even some of the big-name so-called "natural products" are based on petrochemicals. On labels, prefixes or suffixes such as propyl-, methyl-, eth-, or -ene are also usually petroleum-derived compounds.

So, what's wrong with that? By continuing our reliance on petro-chemicals, we are heading down a one-way street to environmental disaster. Globally, we should be focusing on ways of increasing plant growth and decreasing pollution: switching from fossil-fuel-derived ingredients to plant elements is an important (and easy) step in the process. They may be more expensive: naturally derived alternatives can cost up to 10 or even 20 times more than petrochemical ingredients, but the latter are commercially cheap only at the expense of the earth's resources. Equally important is that ingredient costs usually form a small part of the bill paid for a beauty or personal care product – after manufacturing costs, packaging, transportation, and tax.

So look for products that say "free of petrochemicals" or "no petro-chemical ingredients" on the label.

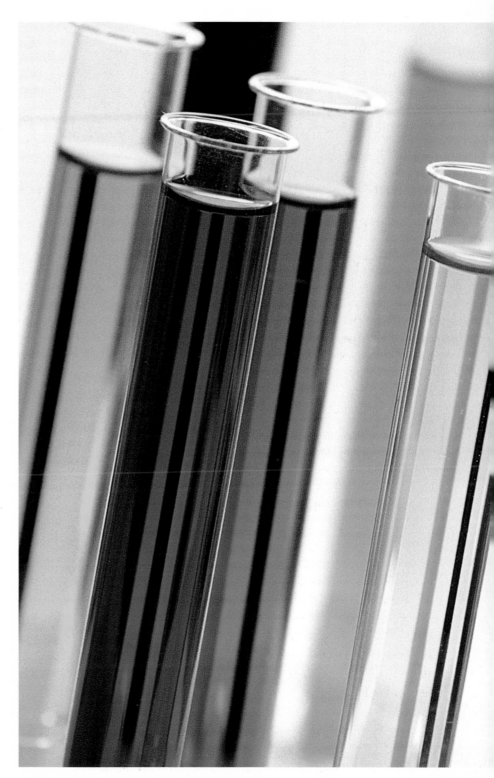

rules for
making your own

When you buy cosmetics, you can seldom be certain *exactly* what has gone into them. Try the following recipes to discover how easy it is to create organic cosmetics in your own kitchen.

In the following pages, you'll find lots of simple recipes for effective alternatives to readymade cosmetics. Few of us have time to rely exclusively on these – just as there are those nights when we reach for pasta and a jar of tomato sauce, or a can of soup, or shove something straight from the freezer into the oven – but it's definitely fun to whoosh up cosmetics yourself, then relax and enjoy the results.

GETTING STARTED

There are some basic rules to assist with making your own cosmetics, and sticking to them will mean that the results don't become contaminated and are "safe" to use.

Just as cooks build up a collection of pots, pans, and utensils for cooking, there is also some useful equipment to sort out before you make your own beauty and bath products, much of which can be found on your saucepan shelf or spoon drawer in the kitchen. If you're going to make your own cosmetics, here is a list of the basic equipment you will require before you start blending.

EQUIPMENT

The following is a list of the equipment that you will need to make organic cosmetics simply and successfully in your own kitchen.

• Egg beater or wire whisk
• Double boiler, or a small saucepan with a Pyrex glass bowl that fits inside to create a double boiler
• Pyrex bowls
• Spoon and cup measures
• Sensitive weighing scales
• Glass dropper (for measuring essential oils)
• Blender or food processor (not essential, it just makes life easier)
• Cheesecloth
• Wire sieve
• Small funnel

Note: Most of the herbs, glycerin, oils, beeswax, and other natural ingredients mentioned in this book can be ordered by mail direct from Neal's Yard Remedies (see *Directory*, pages 122-124). Tincture of benzoin can be bought in a pharmacy, as can witch hazel. Be aware that when you are under stress, your skin may be more sensitive than usual. Perform a skin test, as described on page 19.

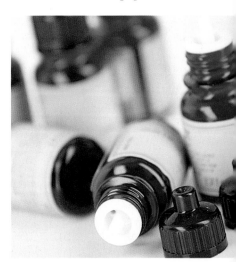

BE SAFE, NOT SORRY

• Choose ingredients that are fresh, pure, and, of course, organic wherever possible. The rule of thumb is: if you wouldn't eat it, don't be tempted to put it on your skin.

• Always use 100 percent pure, unrefined, cold-pressed oils to make sure they are as natural as possible.

• Use your nose: if an oil smells rancid or an ingredient smells strange, do not use it – throw it out.

• Remember, keeping products chilled will extend their shelf life.

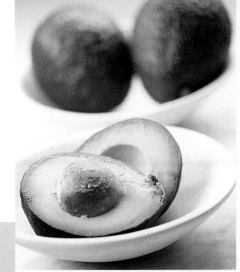

TEST BEFORE YOU USE

Just as you can suffer adverse reactions to readymade cosmetics, so natural, homemade lotions and potions can trigger sensitivity. Avocado oil, essential oils, glycerin, lanolin, simple tincture of benzoin, sweet almond oil, and wheatgerm oil have all been known to cause irritation in some individuals. If you know your skin is particularly sensitive, it is well worth carrying out a patch test before applying any creams to your face or large areas of the body. Here's how:

• Apply a small amount of the substance to your inner arm, immediately below the elbow. Cover with a bandage (unless you're allergic to them), and leave for 24 hours. As an alternative, you could apply the cream behind one ear.

• If any soreness, redness, or irritation occurs, your skin is reacting to an ingredient. It could be one of those listed above, but could also be any ingredient to which you are intolerant. You should determine which ingredient has caused the reaction and avoid using it.

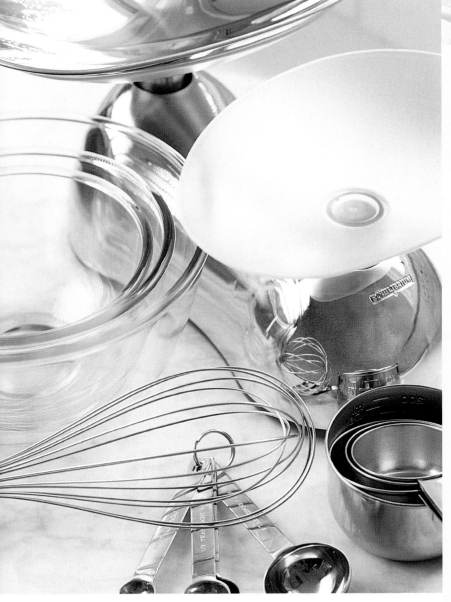

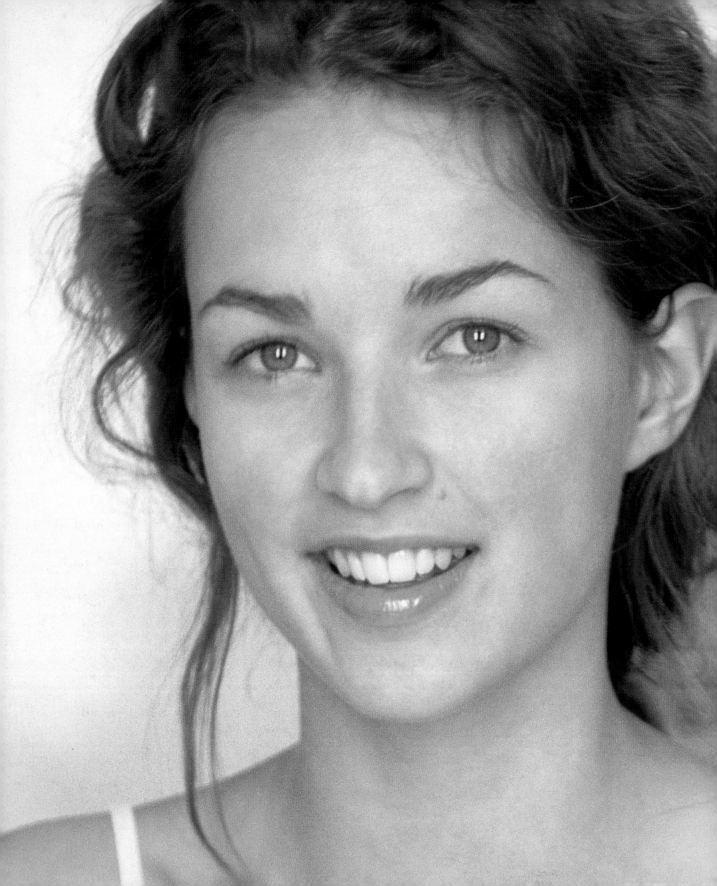

Many women's skincare regimes feature a dozen – or even more – products in the space of a week, designed to keep us squeaky-clean or delay the aging process. One of the key steps to becoming an

Everyday **care**

organic beauty, then, is to simplify your beauty routine. Here's how to find out what your skin really needs – and what it doesn't – at different times of the year and stages of your life. Discover, too, just how simple it is to make 100-percent natural skin treatments – the ultimate in organic beauty.

your skin's *enemies*

In a perfect world, the skin can protect and repair itself extremely well. But in our modern environment, sunlight, pollution, and chemical exposure can cause untold damage.

Each day, the world exerts a certain amount of trauma on your skin. Just as you do your best to adapt to changes that come your way, your skin does its best, too. As you sit at your desk, eat lunch in the park, or walk down the street, your skin is working hard to regulate heat, excrete water and salts as sweat, and provide oxygen to the body. But it is prevented from functioning at its best by routine exposure to environmental stresses. For a healthy, glowing complexion, skin needs to be buffered against potential damage. So, what assaults skin? And what can we do about it?

• **Sun.** 90 percent of premature aging is linked with overexposure to UV rays.

The solution: shield your skin from the sun with any of the natural skin protectors described on page 23.

• **Smoking**. Another skin enemy – even passive smoking. When tobacco burns, as many as 4,000 different chemical compounds are produced: these may be absorbed via your skin. These chemicals affect your internal health, causing lung, heart, blood, and stomach disease, and can cause a variety of visible problems, including skin discoloration or irritation and blackheads. More worryingly, the chemicals can also cause skin cancer.

The solution: creams featuring antioxidant ingredients, such as vitamins C and E, can help protect against – and may even reverse – some of the damage triggered by smoking. If you really can't give up smoking, consider switching to American Spirit cigarettes (available in natural food stores), which are chemical free.

• **Pollution.** Skin can be exposed to hundreds of chemicals a day. According to Toby Mathias, M.D., former head of Occupational Dermatology at the National Institute of Occupational Safety & Health,

"while there are strict regulations regarding the chemicals we breathe or ingest, little is done to restrict the toxins we touch and handle, or that skin comes into direct contact with."

The solution: as a first step, switch to natural cleaning materials. Try the widely available Ecover; or Uniren, Uniclean, and Green Clean, from the Danish company Urtekram. For help sourcing these products see *Directory,* pages 122-124. To protect your skin, also choose body and face creams featuring antioxidant ingredients.

• **Alcohol.** It dehydrates the skin and leads to broken or swollen capillaries, especially on areas of the nose and cheeks. Alochol also destroys the vitamins and minerals needed for a healthy complexion.

The solution: cut down to one or two glasses of good wine a day, and maintain an adequate intake of Essential Fatty Acids (see pages 66-67.)

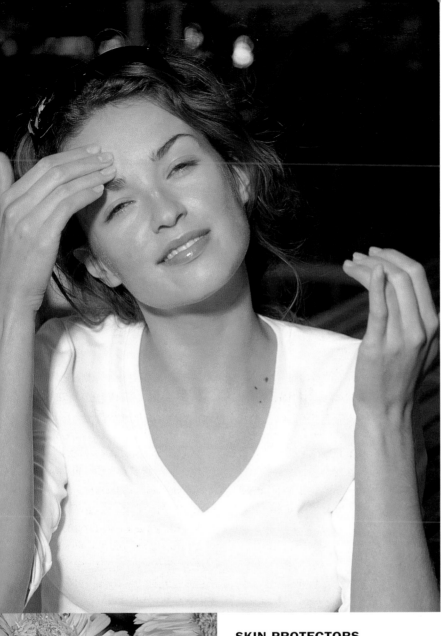

features, the larger the amount that has been used and, therefore, the greater the skin may benefit from the product.

- **Borage oil**, taken from the herb, is an important source of Essential Fatty Acids (see pages 66-67.) EFAs aid in plumping up skin cells and help them retain moisture.
- **Calendula (marigold extract)** helps skin regenerate and heal. It also has an anti-inflammatory action that helps ease skin irritations.
- **Chamomile** has a calming, gentle effect that is good for helping sensitive skin to heal.
- **Lecithin** is an extract from soybeans. It is used to soothe and moisturize skin, and leaves it feeling smooth. Remember: natural beauty companies reject GM soy, whereas many mainstream companies do not (see page 15.)
- **Oatmeal** soothes skin and helps relieve itching and inflammation. It also moisturizes skin and leaves it feeling silky.
- **Vitamin C** helps wounds heal, stimulates collagen, and promotes elastin tissue growth. It also fights free radicals, triggered by sun exposure, pollution, or stress, that can cause damage to skin.
- **Vitamin E** is an antioxidant that helps skin fight sun and smog damage. Look for it on product labels as d-alpha tocopherol, which is the natural form of vitamin E. Alternatively, you could try breaking open a capsule of vitamin E oil and massaging it directly onto your skin.

SKIN PROTECTORS

Sometimes, your skin may be on overload. Life-stress, chemical exposure, UV damage, and many more factors can combine to give skin its own nervous breakdown.

The following list includes some particularly skin-soothing ingredients that you may want to look for when reading cosmetics labels. Remember: the higher up the label the ingredient

avoiding
product overload

Skin experts are agreed that cleansing is actually the most important step in our daily skincare ritual. So here's how to gently cleanse and exfoliate your skin simply and organically.

Most skins are on product overload. Skin has simple needs: to be cleansed, moisturized, nourished, and protected. Despite what the beauty industry tells us, our shelves do not need to groan with creams, lotions, and potions. In fact, some experts believe that the current epidemic of sensitive skin – with 63 percent of women complaining that their skin is more sensitive than normal – can be linked to the unnecessarily complicated beauty regimes touted by cosmetics companies.

Your organic beauty mantra should be: Keep It Simple. Don't apply layer upon layer of products. At a push, you could survive on a single oil alone, such as olive oil or jojoba oil, used both as a cleanser and nourisher (although this is not recommended in the sun because, without protection, you could end up frying your skin.)

Natural beauty brands or homemade cosmetics offer solutions for every skin type and for every age.

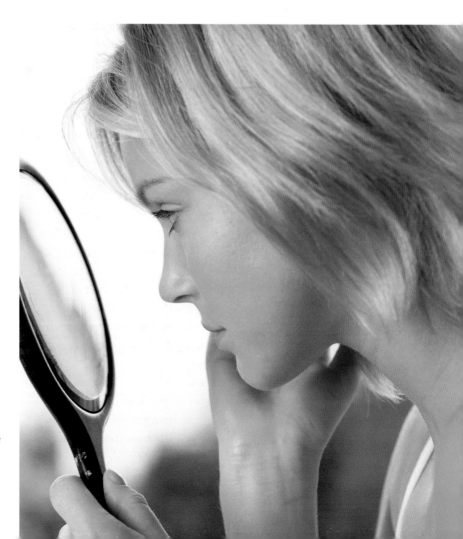

YOUR SKIN TYPE
– AND WHAT IT NEEDS

Oily skin

Do you shine easily? Are your pores large, or does your skin have a sallow cast? If the answer is yes, your skin is almost certainly oily. Console yourself, however, with the knowledge that oily skin tends to age more slowly.

Oily-skinned people, and those who break out in pimples frequently, are often advised to use skin-stripping toners and cleansers. Yet the only effect of these harsh products is to send oil production into turbo-drive. In reality, simplifying and using gentler products is the answer.

What you do need:
• A lightweight, liquid cleanser.
• A skin freshener without alcohol.
• A light moisturizer for drier areas such as your cheeks and neck.
• Sun protection over the whole face when you're gardening, hiking, swimming, or spending large amounts of time outdoors.
• You can enjoy once- or twice-weekly face masks targeted at your skin type, if you like.

What you don't need:
• Harsh, oil-stripping cleansers and facial toners.
• Mattifying or oil-blotting products. To blot your skin, take a facial tissue and separate the layers. Place one layer over the skin and press. It will blot oil without removing your makeup, and can be done as often as you like through the day.

Dry skin

Does your skin peel and flake? Do you have an occasional tendency to redness or sensitive skin? Does it feel tight, as if it's been stretched? Answer "yes" to any of these questions, and your skin is probably dry. Dry skin is lacking in elasticity and has a tendency to wrinkle more. It's also a fact that as we age and oil production slows down naturally, most skins become drier.

What you do need:
• A richer, hydrating cleanser, which can be removed with water or organic cotton balls.
• A nourishing daily moisturizer.
• Facial oils, at night.
• Sun protection, when you're spending time outdoors.
• Once-a-week deep hydrating masks (if you choose).

What you don't need:
• Soap (ever, on your face, and probably only on hands and feet).
• Alcohol-based toners, which are much too harsh for dry skin. If you like to remove every last trace of make-up, use a freshener such as rosewater, or create your own (see pages 30-31.)
• Specific anti-aging creams. Although many may have visible short-term skin-brightening or smoothing effects, nobody yet knows whether, over 20 or 30 years, interfering with the skin's natural mechanisms will produce side-effects, maybe even hastening aging. Organic beauty uses nature's bounty, including time-honored ingredients that have been used to turn back the clock for thousands of years.

Sensitive skin

Is your skin tight, painful, red, itchy, or flaky? Does it come out in occasional bumps, itching, or rashes when you apply creams? It's probably dry and occasionally reactive, or sensitive. This is more common than an allergy, in which a specific ingredient triggers a reaction every time. Treat as dry skin, carry out patch tests on new cosmetics (see page 19,) and try to identify the ingredients that cause problems.

Problem skin

Does your skin have frequent spots, rather than the occasional pimple? Is it reddened and sore? Almost all problem skin is fundamentally oily, so follow the advice for that skin type, and above all, keep your regime simple. Avoid harsh spot creams in favor of natural options that work with the skin. (For more on problem skin, see pages 26-27.)

Combination skin

Many people have skin that is oily in the central T-zone, and dry on the cheeks. Use a cleanser for oily skin, following the advice for that skin type, and use a richer moisturizer for drier skin zones. Many women who complain of having combination skin end up with unnecessarily complicated rituals, when what they're really worried about is the shine on the central panel of their face. In place of mattifying products to mop up shine, try the one-layer-of-tissue trick (see "oily skin," above.)

products
to suit your age

If you are a teenager or a fortysomething plus, your skin needs extra-special care. Follow these recipes using natural oils to give your skin V.I.P. treatment, whatever your age.

Hormones. We can't do without them, but they send skin into turmoil, especially in teenage years and around menopause. When we're in our teens, and sometimes into our twenties, hormones send oil glands into overdrive, triggering overproduction and resulting in shine, pimples, and spots. The conventional beauty industry sells hundreds of millions of dollars' worth of "skin-stripping" cosmetics each year – which all too often worsen the problem they are intended to cure. The more oil that is stripped away, the more skin tries to rebalance itself, by producing even more oil.

HOW TO BEAT HORMONES
Instead of continuing this cycle, your skin regime should become simpler in order to deal with the problems (see pages 24-25). In addition, there are some trouble-shooting natural remedies to help calm and soothe troubled skin.

Mature skin, meanwhile, becomes drier and more papery as estrogen production slows down. It develops crêpiness and wrinkles, because the skin produces less of the lubricating oil that is the curse of so many teenagers. Added to this, the barrier function – the protective role of skin – becomes less effective with age; as skin becomes thinner, it is easier for moisture to escape. That is why dry skin is increasingly a problem as we age. To tackle dry skin in your daily regime, follow the guidelines on page 25.

The anti-aging skincare industry is worth millions if not billions of dollars. However, it will be years before the long-term effects of some of the ingredients, for instance, fruit acids (which work by exfoliating the skin's top layers, on a daily basis), are seen and truly understood. Will these anti-aging preparations actually speed up the march of time, or will they turn back the clock as promised? So far,

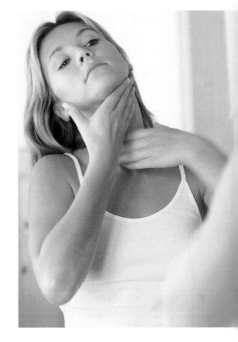

nobody knows. But certainly, the organic beauty world has plenty of natural anti-agers to help skin retain its youthful glow – such as frankincense oil. On the following page are some skin "treats" that should help put back what the years take out.

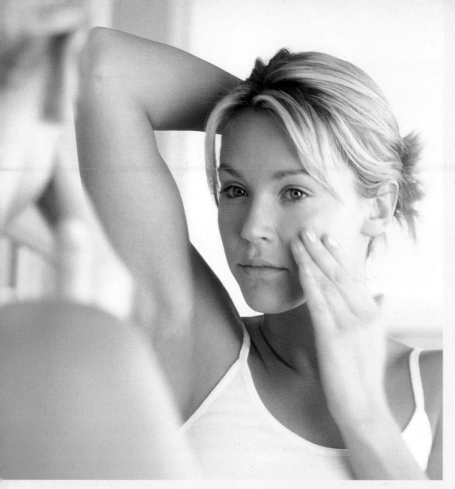

Combine all the oils and keep in a dark glass jar with a dropper top. Massage a single drop into the area of the orbital bone around the eye at night; use more generously on the neck area.

Calendula balm for sensitive skin

1 oz (25 g) calendula blossoms
½ cup extra virgin olive oil
1 oz (25 g) beeswax

Using a mortar and pestle (or an electronic herb grinder), grind the calendula blossoms and place them in the bottom of a glass jar. Pour in the olive oil, and allow the mixture to steep. Shake daily for about three weeks, when you'll have a wonderful soothing oil base for the sensitive balm. Strain through a fine cloth into a bowl, squeezing and pressing until the last drops are filtered.

To make the balm itself, place a heat-proof glass measuring cup in a pan containing about 4 in (10 cm) of water, and warm over a medium heat. Put the oil base and then the grated beeswax into the cup and stir with a chopstick or wooden spoon until thoroughly melted. Pour the mixture into wide-mouthed jars, then let it cool and solidify.

To test the consistency, drop a small amount onto a saucer and put it in the freezer for one minute. If you want a harder balm, add a little beeswax. If the balm is too hard, add a little oil to soften up the balm. (Hot weather makes a difference, too; you may need more beeswax when it's warm outside.) Store away from heat and light. Apply whenever skin is inflamed or sore.

Facial oil for oily skin

¼ cup (50 ml) grapeseed oil
2 tbs jojoba oil
8 drops cedarwood oil
10 drops lemon oil
5 drops ylang-ylang oil

Mix all the oils. Then tie your hair off your face, and with clean hands, massage the oil into the skin. This blend will help regulate the skin's natural oil production.

Oil for problem skin

¼ cup (50 ml) apricot oil
10 drops lemon oil
10 drops cypress oil
5 drops lavender oil

Combine the oils and massage well into the area of lymph glands (down both sides of the neck), the sinus area, and the forehead. Pouring oil on troubled skin – in which oil production is already in overdrive – might not sound logical, but if you persist with daily treatments using this treatment oil for acne, you should see benefits. (It is possible that the oil tricks the skin into believing it has produced enough oil and so slows down production.)

Replenishing neck and eye oil for mature skin

1½ tsp glycerin
¼ cup (50 ml) apricot kernel oil
30 drops jojoba oil
3 drops neroli oil
2 drops ylang-ylang oil
2 drops frankincense oil

cleansing *and toning*

Skin experts are agreed that cleansing and toning are actually the most important steps in our skincare ritual. So here's how to create a simple and organic skincare routine.

Many cleansers on the market contain ingredients such as mineral oil and petrolatum; they may be excellent at removing makeup and grime but are anything but ecofriendly. Their basic ingredient is mined from fossil deposits; it's the same oil that goes in our cars, but refined differently. These ingredients also sit on the surface and block pores, sometimes leading to little white pimples under the skin or to other types of spots. Mineral oil is also used as a moisturizing ingredient because it creates an occlusive barrier that actually traps the skin's own natural moisture.

As an alternative to these products, look in natural food stores for more natural cleansers. Lines such as Dr. Hauschka and Jurlique offer unusual alternatives in the form of oatmeal-based pastes, which some famous beauties swear by, although they are quite messy to use.

FACE FACTS

Soap, even handmade soap, is too harsh for facial skin, upsetting its acid balance (pH), so the skin feels taut and tight. If you like to use water, there are plenty of other options to soap or beauty bars. Oily skins respond best to lotion-type cleansers, whereas dry and sensitive skins love oil-based cleansers (see page 30 for recipes.)

Nature provides superb alternatives to commercial cleansers: oils, which literally melt makeup and pollution from your face. Now that organic oils are more widely available, it is easy to create 100-percent organic cleansers of your own. Any nut or seed oil can be used to massage and cleanse the face.

If you cleanse properly, you really don't need a toner. Contrary to myth, toners cannot "close" pores – because they do not physically open and shut in the first place. What toners can do is create a sensation of freshness, which is why some women still love the feel of them. If you do want to use a toner, choose one that's alcohol-free: alcohol overstrips the skin and upsets

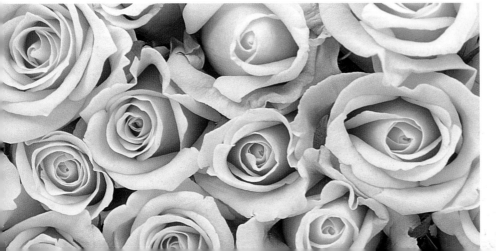

its vital natural oil balance. The word "freshener" (instead of "toner") can be a clue that a product is alcohol-free, but to be certain, check the ingredient list. Rosewater and orange flower water, both widely available, make alternative face refreshers. (Try spritzing them on with a pump-action spray, rather than using cotton balls; you can also use this to set makeup.) Or make your own fresheners: you're about to discover how easy that is.

COTTON ONTO ORGANIC

Cotton is the most heavily sprayed crop on the planet (cocoa comes second.) So if you buy regular cotton balls, not only do traces of those pesticides inevitably end up on your face, but you're contributing to one of the world's most polluting forms of agriculture. Organic cotton balls are increasingly widely available (even in supermarkets): just as soft and just as effective, but this cotton really is as pure as it looks.

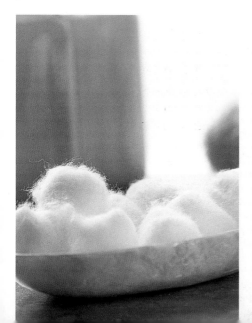

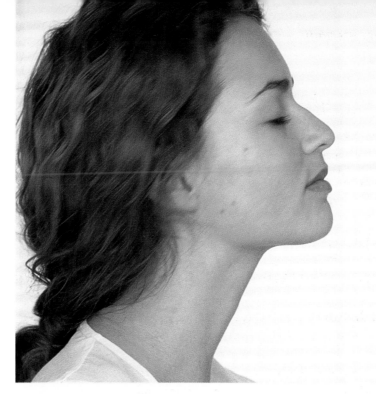

STARTING AFRESH

Cleansing is a blissful end-of-day ritual that helps relax the body and mind before sleeping. You can enhance it by using a little creative visualization: imagine, as you wipe away the buildup of toxins, sweat, and cosmetics from your face, that you are literally melting away the day's anxieties and worries and sending them down the sink.

The cleansed face that you're left with is like a smooth canvas, a blank page – literally, a fresh start.

THE ULTIMATE CLEANSE

The very best way to remove makeup is not with facial tissues (even recycled ones) or cotton balls – it's with pieces of cheesecloth. You can either buy these readymade (see *Directory,* pages 122-124), or make your own with 100-percent natural cheesecloth bought in a fabric or department store. Cut it into squares measuring roughly 12 in (30 cm).

To use the cloth, simply apply your cleanser and massage it thoroughly into your face. Soak the cloth in hot water and use it like a washcloth to remove every last trace of cleanser. Rinse the cloth and repeat two or three times; then finish by running it under a cool faucet and wiping that over your face.

Hang the cloth over a radiator or the edge of the bathtub to dry; this will help guarantee that bacteria don't get the chance to breed in the cloth. Every couple of days, switch to a fresh piece of cloth.

The cheesecloth squares can be washed in a washing machine, with "green" detergent, or boiled in a saucepan with a drop of bleach. They can be used again and again.

making
skincare products

You, better than anyone, know your skin's likes and dislikes, so why opt for commercial products when you can make your own at home, using exactly what your skin type desires?

Cleopatra's cleansing oil

This cleanser has a useful antimicrobial action, and it is also fantastic for dissolving and removing makeup.

⅛ cup (25 ml) olive oil

¼ cup (50 ml) grapeseed oil

⅛ cup (25 ml) coconut oil

7 drops rosemary essential oil

6 drops orange essential oil

4 drops tea tree essential oil

3 drops sage essential oil

Place a heatproof measuring cup inside a saucepan of water that has recently boiled. Pour the coconut oil into the cup and heat until the oil has completely melted. Blend in the other oils. Pour the mixture into a squeeze bottle or a wide-mouthed jar, stirring well. Then put on the top and shake. As it cools, it will thicken slightly.

Simple cleansing cream

Like most readymade cleansers, this cream is a mix of oil and water. It's light to use and effective. It is suitable for all skin types, but particularly oily or normal.

¼ oz (5 g) beeswax

½ cup (100 ml) grapeseed oil

⅔ cup (120 ml) distilled or spring water

½ tsp borax powder

12 drops rosemary essential oil (optional)

8 drops lavender essential oil (optional)

5 drops orange essential oil (optional)

Place the beeswax and the grapeseed oil in a heatproof measuring cup in a recently boiled saucepan of water. Stir occasionally until the wax has melted entirely into the oil. Remove from the heat and let it cool to body temperature. Next, warm the distilled or spring water to body temperature and dissolve the ½ tsp of borax powder in it. Pour the wax and oil mixture into a bowl and add the water and borax mixture a little at a time, beating it with a hand-held mixer until it reaches a creamy, thick consistency (this should take about five minutes to reach the right consistency.) If you want to add the essential oils, do so now. Stir the mixture until the oils have blended thoroughly.

Richer cleansing cream

⅛ cup (25 ml) jojoba oil

⅛ cup (25 ml) grapeseed oil

½-1 oz (10-20 g) beeswax (use less for a thinner cream)

¼ cup (50 ml) lavender water or rosewater

1 tsp vegetable glycerin

1 tsp borax

Antioxidant preservative: either 1 tsp vitamin C powder, ¼ tsp vitamin A powder, or 1 tsp of wheatgerm oil

10 drops of essential oil (rose or lavender)

Melt the beeswax into the oils in a double boiler placed over medium heat. When melted, remove the mixture from the heat and pour in all the other ingredients. Mix with an electric hand-held mixer until it reaches a thick, creamy consistency.

For cleansing, apply the cream to your face with your fingers, massage in well all over your face and neck, and rinse well with warm water. This rich cleansing cream works particularly well on mature and dry skin types.

Soothing skin tonic

3 tbs dried or fresh
   marigold leaves
2½ cups (500 ml) spring water
1 tbs apple juice

Place the leaves in a bowl, boil the spring
water, and pour it on the leaves. Steep for
20 minutes. Add the apple juice; pour into
a sterilized bottle and let it cool.

Lavender freshener for oily or problem skins

1 cup (200 ml) witch hazel
15 drops lavender oil

Combine the ingredients and store in
a pretty bottle (use one with a spray
top if it is to be used as a spritzer).
Apply either with a cotton pad, or by
spritzing onto the face after cleansing.

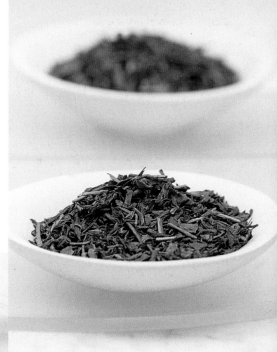

Green tea toner

This is rich in antioxidants, which are
believed to have an anti-aging effect not
only when taken internally, but also when
applied to the skin.

1 cup (200 ml) spring water
4 tsp green tea leaves
1 tsp mint leaves

Boil the spring water and make an
infusion with the leaves. Let it stand for
10 minutes. Strain the infusion and let the
liquid cool before pouring it into a
sterilized bottle. Apply to the face with a
cotton pad, or use as a spritz.

Because this toner does not contain any
alcohol, it's also suitable for dry and
sensitive skins.

It is rich in antioxidants, which are
believed to have an anti-aging effect when
applied to the skin. Green tea is one of
the "buzz" ingredients recently discovered
by the skincare industry, and this simple
freshener is the ultimate way to give your
skin a "drink" of green tea.

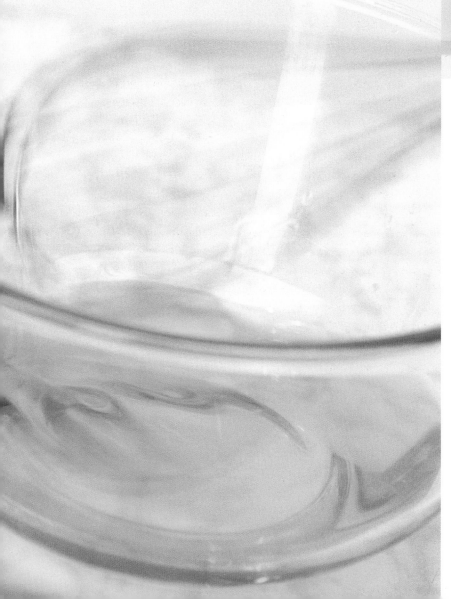

hydrating
the skin

The dry air generated by central heating and air-conditioning, and exposure to the elements can dehydrate our skin. Nourish your skin by replenishing the water it loses every day.

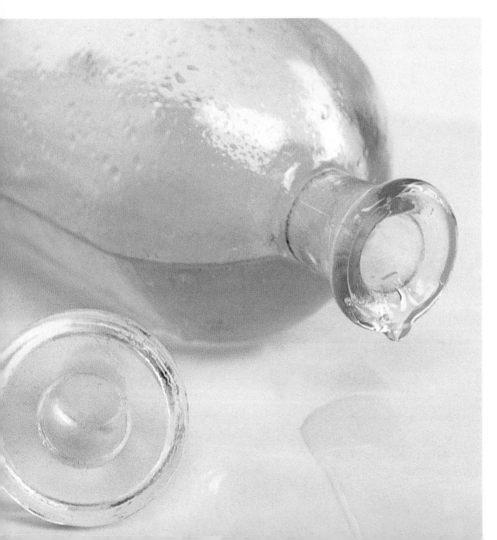

Skin is thirsty; it craves oil and moisture. Oil keeps it supple and moisture plumps up the skin cells, making them look younger. Without these two elements, skin begins to sag and wrinkle, and it feels unpleasantly taut and dry. That is why every branded moisturizer on the market is basically a mixture of oil and water, blended with emulsifiers to keep them from separating, which they would do naturally after a very short time.

The problem with emulsifiers, however, is that many of them create problems for sensitive skin. Instead of sitting on the skin's surface, emulsifiers make inroads into the outer skin barrier so irritants, essential oils, and other chemicals can get below the surface. Here, they may set off a reaction, seen on the skin as redness or bumps, and felt as itching or burning. Making your own creams avoids the need for emulsifiers, since you can maintain fresh supplies and remix if the cream separates.

WHAT TO AVOID

If you buy over-the-counter moisturizers, avoid pore-blocking ingredients such as petrolatum and mineral oil. Look among the natural brands for products with short ingredient lists, which indicates that fewer preservatives and chemicals have been used in their preparation. Logona, Weleda, Dr. Hauschka, Jurlique, and Burt's Bees are among the brands that offer 100-percent natural, synthetic-chemical-free skincare. Alternatively, make your own.

FACIAL CREAMS AND OILS

By day wear a cream, as protection and as a smooth base for makeup. At night, experiment with facial oils: pure, liquid plant energy. Many facial oils have a hazelnut oil base, a featherlight plant oil to which is added wheatgerm, grapeseed, and active essential oils, with maybe a little antioxidant vitamin E. Other facial oils may be created with wheatgerm, grapeseed, or almond oil bases.

These facial oils sink into the skin surprisingly fast and, provided "balancing" essential oils are used, can work even for oily skins (oil doesn't need to make oily skin greasy.) Find beautiful blends in lines by Decléor, E'SPA, Aesop, Clarins, Neal's Yard, Elemis, Dr. Hauschka, Caudalie, Cariad, and Jurlique. Alternatively, have the reassurance of knowing that what you're feeding your face is 100-percent organic, by making your own moisturizing creams and oils.

Basic moisturizer

¼ oz (5 g) beeswax

2 tbs almond oil

1½ tbs spring water or rosewater

4 drops essential oil – rose or frankincense for dry or aging skin; lavender for normal skin; lemon for oily/combination skin

1 tsp wheatgerm oil (a natural preservative)

Melt the beeswax and the oil in a heatproof bowl over a pan of simmering water, or use a double boiler. Heat the water in another double boiler or bowl over a pan of simmering water until warm. Add the warm water to the oil and wax using a dropper, drop by drop, beating with a whisk. When you have mixed 1 tsp of the water with the oil and beeswax, remove the pan from the heat and add all the other ingredients. Pour into a sterile jar and cool; refrigerate to maintain freshness. The cream softens on contact with the skin.

Ultra-rich moisturizer

4 tbs avocado oil

4 tbs wheatgerm oil

1 oz (25 g) cocoa butter

1 tsp beeswax

½ tsp borax powder

2 tbs rosewater

10 drops geranium essential oil

5 drops frankincense essential oil

5 drops sandalwood essential oil

Put the wheatgerm and avocado oil together in a heatproof bowl and place in a saucepan half-full of water. Add the cocoa butter and the beeswax, and heat until the mixture is completely blended and smooth. Dissolve the borax in the rosewater and add to the waxy mixture on the stove. Stir thoroughly, remove from the heat, and add the essential oils. Keep stirring until it is cool enough to pour into a sterilized glass jar with a lid.

FACIAL OILS FOR ALL SKINTYPES

For dry skin: Mix 4 drops each of geranium and chamomile essential oil and 2 drops each of lemon and lavender oil into 2 tablespoons sweet almond oil. This perfectly moisturizes even sore and chapped skin.

For oily skin, problem skin, and mature skin, see the products to suit your skintype and facial oil recipes outlined on page 27.

working

with nature

The sun provides us with energy and light. The moon exerts its influence on the tides and our own monthly cycle. Find out how to become a lunar beauty – and play safe in the sun.

One day, cosmetics may not need preservatives – if manufacturers are prepared to make them according to lunar cycles. Dr. Hauschka's bio-dynamic skincare has always been made in rhythm with the moon, and Gaby Just, a German beauty who now has her own cosmetics line, Just Pure (see *Directory,* pages 122-124), has also discovered the potent effect of the moon while creating her products. Struggling to make preservative-free cosmetics that had a shelf-life, Gaby Just found that they didn't develop bacteria or molds when she made them at certain times in the lunar cycle. This led her to research the moon's impact on our skin, body, and psyche as well.

LUNAR BEAUTY

Have you ever wondered why a bikini wax is sometimes agony and yet at other times it is almost pain-free? Or why, occasionally, you have a non-PMS-linked food craving? In fact, just as biodynamic gardening recognizes the impact of the moon's phases on growing cycles, so the moon affects our body's functions, too. Keep a lunar calendar on your desk and start to observe the link for yourself.

• The waxing moon is a time of regenerating and absorbing. Everything applied to the skin in the 12 days of the waxing moon has a much greater effect, so it's the best time for aromatic oil massages, nourishing treatments, and masks.

• At full moon, skin seems to be at its most absorbent, so facial oils, herb compresses, or oil baths have an optimum effect. If you have only a little time each month for a pampering blitz, make it now.

• A waning moon is a good time to start a diet, or an anticellulite program, especially skin-brushing.

• New moon is when purification and detoxifying are at their most effective. It's a great time for a juice or tea fast.

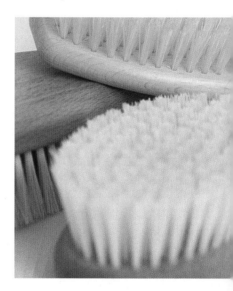

• The best time for hair waxing, or for getting your teeth fixed, is at new moon or under a waning moon, when you'll experience the least pain. The opposite is true at full moon.

• If you're going to grow your own herbs in the garden or a windowbox for making masks or for aromatherapy treatments, the best time to pick them is full moon.

SUN: THE BURNING TRUTH

For years, suncare manufacturers have been telling us to slather on Sun Protection Factors (SPF) in the sun, "safe" in the knowledge that the chemical and reflective ingredients in the product multiplies our natural

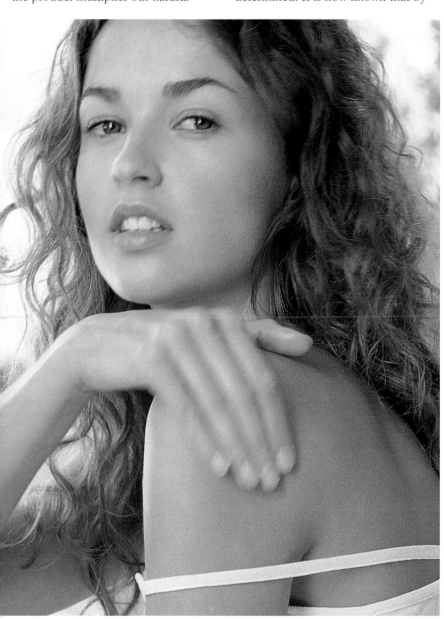

protection by 8, 10, 25, 30, or more – depending on the SPF figure on the front of the packaging. Real life, however, turns out to be quite different from the laboratory conditions under which SPFs are determined. It is now known that by

the time you've massaged cream into your skin, the protection it delivers is about a third to one-half of that figure promised on the packaging. This does not suggest that we should stop using sunscreens – only that, to be safe, we should rely on sunscreens as part of a more fully structured "safe sun" strategy (see page 36).

Because, in summer, we slather on so many products to shield the skin from UV light, finding truly natural suncare is high on the organic shopper's priority list. This is easier said than done, since many sunscreen products advertised as "natural" actually contain the same active chemical ingredients as mainstream brands.

Chemical sunscreens, which absorb light, are popular because they are invisible and long-lasting – however, they are also a cocktail of chemicals whose trouble-triggering potential is supercharged by sitting in the sun. This is why they are linked with skin sensitivity in many sunbathers.

Become a label-scanner and avoid harsh chemical ingredients. These include PABA (para-amino-benzoic acid) and the benzophenones, such as benzophenone-3 and oxybenzone, together with cinnamates (such as octyl methoxycinnamate and methoxy cinnamate) and salicylates (such as octyl salicylate).

Another downside of chemical ingredients is that, ironically, they tend to start breaking down and becoming less effective just as soon as they have been exposed to the sun!

sun
protection

Sunshine improves your mental health dramatically, but it can have devastating physical effects. Make sure that you are properly protected so you can enjoy the sun's benefits safely.

Wearing sunblock is like wearing thousands of tiny mirrors on the skin that reflect back the sun's rays. They sit on top of the skin and so are less irritating than sunscreens. The ingredients to look for are titanium dioxide and zinc oxide, which are milled from minerals. In the old days, they gave skin a white or gray cast, but new micro-milling techniques mean they're almost invisible on skin while offering optimum protection.

Alas, it isn't possible to make your own sunscreens safely. However, a couple of companies make sun protection based on mineral sunblock ingredients: Dr. Hauschka and Weleda. Jurlique uses a tiny percentage of chemical sunscreens, holding the opinion that the tradeoff between a very small amount of chemicals for a more effective product is worth it.

In addition to using sunblock, protect skin naturally from within by eating a good wholefood diet, with plenty of brightly colored vegetables and fruits, which are naturally protective. Take supplements of antioxidant vitamins A (such as beta-carotene), C, and E to boost that protection (ask about quantities at your natural food store), and above all, use common sense. Drink plenty of spring water, too, to prevent the skin from dehydrating.

THE SPF OF TREES

Who needs sunscreen when there are trees? Trees offer great SPF. Even in their shade, you'll pick up a little color, but more healthily and slowly. Research shows that an oak tree provides an SPF of 10-20; an elm or a maple offers SPF30; and a dense pine forest gives SPF100.

SMART SUNNING

• When shopping, you need to be aware that the actual SPF rating of your sun cream is likely to be between one-half and one-third of the SPF stated on the packaging.

• Never sunbathe – you'll pick up some color just by walking around, even from lying in the shade.

• Avoid sun exposure during the peak hours: between 10 a.m. and 3 p.m.

• Be sunsmart even on cloudy days: UV rays can penetrate clouds, and the aging UVA rays in sunlight can even go through glass.

• The sun's rays are more intense in tropical and semitropical locations, because exposure becomes more direct the closer you get to the equator. Intensity is also increased in higher elevations where the atmosphere is thinner. Extra protection for eyes and lips is necessary, in both cases.

• Apply sunscreen 15 to 30 minutes before you go outdoors, and let it dry or bond with the skin before dressing. Apply again as soon as you are in direct sunlight: you can burn just while looking for a recliner or a place to have a picnic.

• Protect yourself while swimming, and reapply afterward.

• You can cut down on overall exposure received by spending intermittent periods of time in the shade, but be aware that you need to wear sun protection there, too.

• Wear a hat with a four-inch-wide brim (minimum) and sunglasses, even when walking short distances. Sunglasses should also contain UV-protective lenses.

• Cover up. Tightly woven clothing offers the better protection. Loose, tight-weave clothing is best of all.

• Infants under 12 months old should be shielded from any sun exposure. Use an SPF25 or above on children of all ages, and dress them in protective clothing, making sure the ultra-vulnerable back of the neck is well protected. The Skin Cancer Foundation has concluded that if a child is protected from the sun by a high SPF (25-50) at six months, continuing through adolescence, the chances of sun damage or developing skin cancer are greatly reduced.

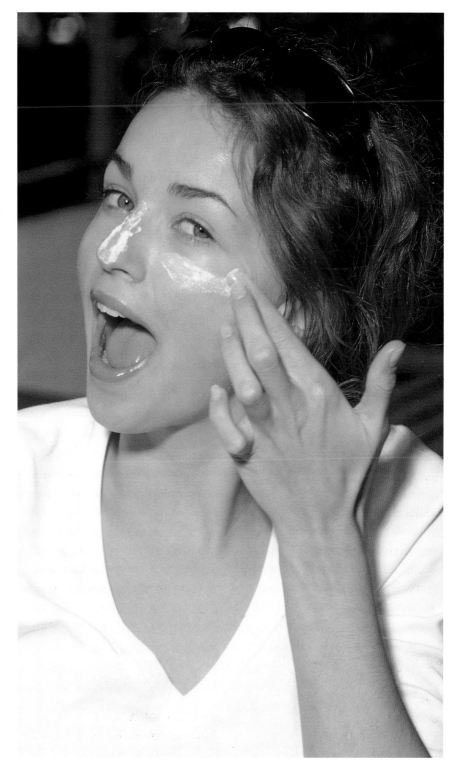

remedies

for burns and bites

At times, we all suffer from over-exposure to the sun – and to insects. Soothe the pain with 100-percent organic remedies from the pantry and let your skin feel healthy again.

Sometimes, accidents happen, and we get sunburned. Nature, however, has plenty of wonderful skin-soothers that can take away the redness and soreness. To tackle burns, not just sunburn but any minor burns, every home should have an *Aloe vera* plant. The plant is not only attractive to look at, but it also harnesses amazing powers.

Aloe cools and soothes even the most tender skin and creates a natural protective bandage as it dries. Doctors in ancient Egypt prescribed aloe for wounds and other skin problems, and Cleopatra rubbed aloe gel into her skin as a beauty treatment. More recently, clinical studies have shown that fresh aloe gel speeds up the healing of wounds and burns, and also fights the bacteria that cause infection.

In hot climates, aloe can be grown outdoors. If you live in a cooler climate, or anywhere where there's a risk of frost, the plant is happiest situated on a table near a window.

To use, simply slice off a leaf of aloe and peel it, then apply to sunburned skin (it leaves a sticky "snail's trail" of soothing gel.) Alternatively, make a batch of aloe vera antioxidant gel and keep it chilled in the refrigerator for use in summer.

To make the gel:
• Slice off a large outer leaf and peel it with a potato peeler or a paring knife. Put it in a blender or food processor.
• For every ¼ cup (50 ml) of aloe gel, add 500 mg of powdered vitamin C, the contents of one vitamin E capsule (400 IU), and ½ tsp lavender essential oil.
• Blend thoroughly. Then apply the gel as needed to cuts, burns, insect bites, and any type of skin irritation. Kept refrigerated in a clean glass jar, this gel will stay fresh for a couple of months.

Recent studies have also shown that slathering skin with extra-virgin olive oil after sun exposure may protect against skin cancer. In tests, skin treated with extra-virgin olive oil after

being blasted with damaging ultraviolet rays developed smaller, fewer, and less life-threatening tumors, probably due to the high level of antioxidants in the oil. So, treat your skin to organic extra-virgin olive oil as an after-sun massage, but be aware that non-virgin olive oil does not offer the same skin protection.

Another effective skin soother is natural yogurt.

BUZZ OFF – NATURALLY
Organic living means avoiding pest sprays on your food. So why on earth would you want to spray them on your skin? Millions of people do just that, however, in an attempt to keep mosquitoes and other bugs at bay.

Ironically, the result of this spraying is that the pests themselves are becoming more resistant, and humans are required to cover themselves in ever stronger chemicals to counteract it. Every generation of pesticides has

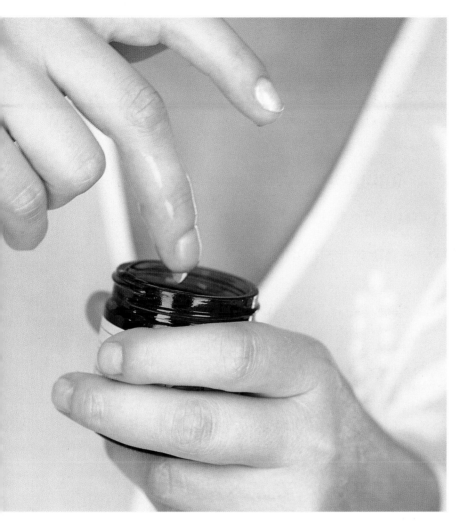

them away from us. For those of us who believe in an ecosystem in which nature's balance is to be maintained, that's a more acceptable approach.

Lavender, geranium, lemon, lemon grass, and citronella essential oils all help repel insects. Vaporize any of them in a burner where you're sitting or sleeping. Alternatively, lavender can be applied undiluted to the skin; the other oils can be diluted in a carrier oil, such as jojoba or grapeseed: to each tablespoon of base oil, add 12 drops of essential oils, and apply to vulnerable areas, especially ankles and wrists.

Neem oil (from the Indian tree *Azadirachta indica*) is said to provide significant protection from mosquitoes for up to 12 hours. Dr. Hauschka makes an oil based on neem.

If indoor bugs are a problem, try hanging strips of cotton cloth that have been dotted with drops of essential oils around the house. In addition to being environmentally friendly, this is also a healthy alternative to chemically treated commercial no-pest strips, some of which have been linked to cancer.

A lavender- or cedar-scented handkerchief, laid in a drawer or tied around a coat hanger, will help keep moths away.

INSECT BITE SOOTHER
If you do get bitten, try a cold compress to calm the area: soak a cloth in ice water to which a few drops of chamomile and lavender oil have been added, then wring out the cloth and lay it on the affected area for 15 minutes.

produced pests with greater resistance.

What's more, some "personal pesticides" appear to have some very unpleasant effects. DEET (*diethyl toluamide*), which was developed for and tested by American troops in the Vietnam War, has triggered adverse reactions in consumers, and there's even a suggestion of a link with infant deaths. In 1989, the Environmental Protection Agency issued a consumer bulletin in response to several reports of headaches, convulsions, and

unconsciousness in people who had used DEET. The bulletin advised people never to use it on irritated or cut skin, to keep it away from the eyes and mouth, and to wash exposed skin with soap and water.

Instinctively, many of us understand that there is absolutely no need to resort to this chemical weaponry against creepy-crawlies. Natural essential oils can help keep them at bay instead. In addition, the oils don't actually kill the bugs – they just keep

reviving
face masks

Face masks are a luxurious addition to your skin routine, making you feel well and truly pampered. Every one of these recipes uses ingredients that are good enough to eat.

Masks are an optional part of a beauty regime; however, many women find that a once- or twice-weekly face mask not only enhances and brightens the complexion, it also provides the perfect excuse to do absolutely nothing for a few peaceful minutes. Best of all, the ingredients for all these recipes can be found effortlessly in your kitchen.

Brightening mask for face and hands

½ avocado

1 tbs tomato pulp

1 tbs lemon juice

Mash the skinned and stoned avocado with the other ingredients until you have a very smooth paste. Spread it over the face, neck, and hands and leave for 20 minutes before washing off with warm water. Pat the skin dry.

For skin that is very dehydrated, use only 1 tbs of lemon juice and omit the tomato pulp. In its place substitute 1 tbs of honey.

Honey and avocado mask for normal-to-dry skin

Eggs and avocado blend beautifully together, and they are both highly moisturizing – avocadoes have a 20 percent fat content. What's more, this recipe uses mayonnaise, which is well known to tone and smooth skin. In an emergency, you can spoon it straight from the jar onto your face!

1 egg

½ avocado (peeled, with the stone taken out)

1 tsp organic mayonnaise

1 tsp honey

1 tsp baking soda

2 drops orange essential oil

Purée the avocado, egg, and mayonnaise in a blender, then add the honey and remaining ingredients. Alternatively, you can beat it by hand, adding the baking soda last.

This mask needs to be used all at once, so apply any extra mixture to the chest and neck areas.

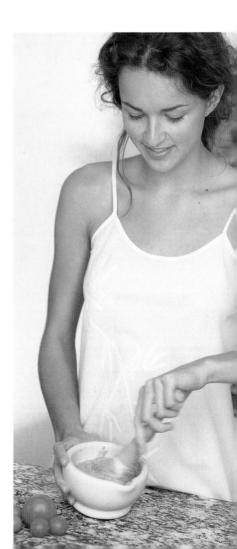

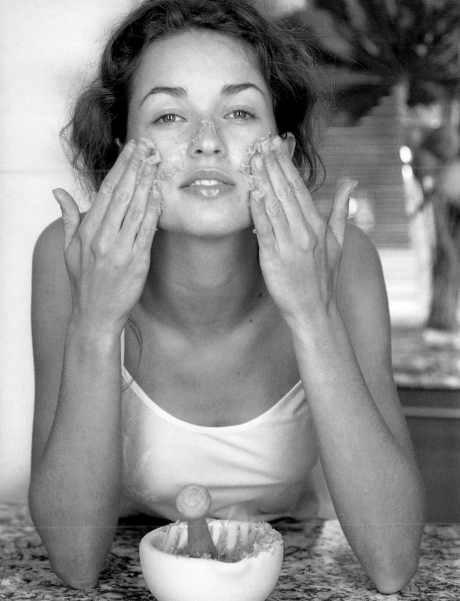

Mask for saggy necks

1 tbs honey
2 tbs almond oil

Mix the ingredients together and gently brush the mixture onto the neck, using a pastry brush. Leave on for 30 minutes, then rinse off with warm water.

Apply this luxurious mask to your neck once a week, and you should notice an ongoing improvement in softness and smoothness.

Keep the mixture in the refrigerator between treatments; if it needs softening before use, dip the jar in an ovenproof bowl of hot water.

French women, in particular, swear by massaging the neck using upward strokes that work against gravity. For the best results, use this method when applying neck creams and oils.

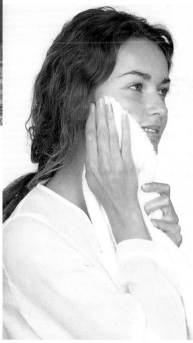

Antiwrinkle mask

1 large carrot
1 tbs olive or almond oil

Grate the carrot, using the grater attachment on your food processor. When it is ready, add the oil and process until combined. Put the mixture in the refrigerator for 1 to 2 hours. Apply around the eyes and cheeks, and leave on for 30 minutes: lie back with your eyes closed and relax. Wipe away with warm water.

Oily skin mask

1 egg white
¼ tsp lemon juice or
**   cider vinegar**

This recipe is so simple and takes just seconds to make. Whisk the egg white, add the lemon juice or cider vinegar, and apply at once to a well-cleansed face. Wash off after 10 minutes.

Don't worry that the mask feels quite tight on the skin: that's normal.

toning
massage

Is your face looking tired? Does it feel in need of a lift? If so, a simple, 12-point pressure massage can help to stimulate the circulation and put back the natural glow and vitality.

"Firming" and "lifting" may be buzzwords in the skincare world at the moment, but the best way to revive a tired, sagging face is not by slapping on a cream. From ancient times, the Japanese and Chinese have used pressure-point techniques to awaken and restore the face, helping to reduce puffiness by improving lymph drainage and stimulating the flow of Chi, the body's vital life energy.

HOW IT WORKS

Facial massage helps defy age by reducing muscle tension – tension that can eventually etch lines in the face. By increasing blood circulation, it brings oxygen and essential nutrients to the skin and helps remove toxins.

Ideally, this facial acupressure-based massage should take 12 minutes, but even a few seconds spent on each acupressure point will make a difference to skin vibrancy.

To get yourself into the routine, try incorporating a massage into your nightly cleansing regime: apply cleanser, massage the facial acupressure points, then wash or remove your cleanser as normal.

A facial massage can be done on bare or made-up skin. On bare skin, a facial massage oil helps the fingers glide from pressure-point to pressure-point. If you are wearing makeup, however, don't skim the fingers over the surface. Take a shiatsu approach and apply fingers to pressure points only. Using the middle finger of each hand, massage the points on each side of the face which mirror each other. For those few acupressure points that are in the center of the face, use the middle finger of either hand.

If you have time, massage each pressure point for up to one minute. Otherwise, using this pressure-point technique for just five or 10 seconds on each area will help.

Step-by-step facial acupressure

1 Locate the spots at the hairline that are directly above the center of the eyes. Massage using inward circles, breathing deeply.

2 Move fingers down the face to half-way between eyebrows and hairline. Massage using inward circles.

3 Use your thumbs for this one: locate the spot on each side of the bridge of the nose, just below the brow line. Push upward, using pressure rather than circling technique. (Note: this can hurt!)

4 At the outer tip of the eyebrows, massage with outward circles.

5 At the outside corner of the eyes, massage outward.

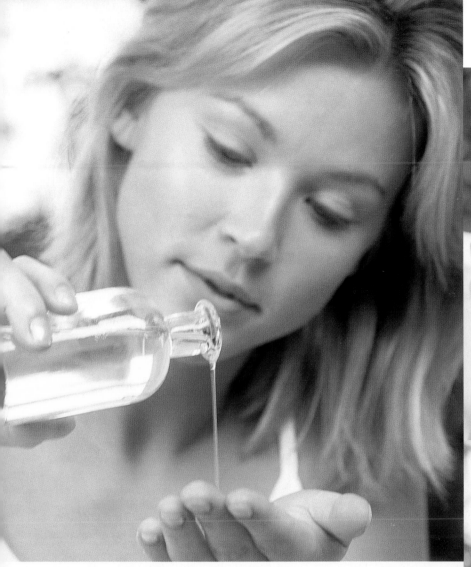

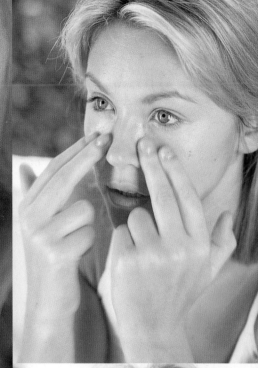

6 On the top of the cheekbone, underneath the middle of the eye, circle outward.

7 Now move the fingers down until they are in line with your nostrils, and massage using outward circles.

8 In the indentation that runs from the middle of your nose to your top lip, circle in a clockwise direction, using one finger.

9 Locate the middle of your chin and massage in clockwise circles.

10 Using both fingers again, place your fingers on the jawline at each side of the chin. Massage in outward circles.

11 Move your fingers outward along the jaw to a point halfway between jaw and the jaw hinge. Massage in outward circles.

12 Find the muscle just in front of the jaw hinge (there'll be a slight indentation). With the mouth resting open, massage the area by making circles toward the back of the head.

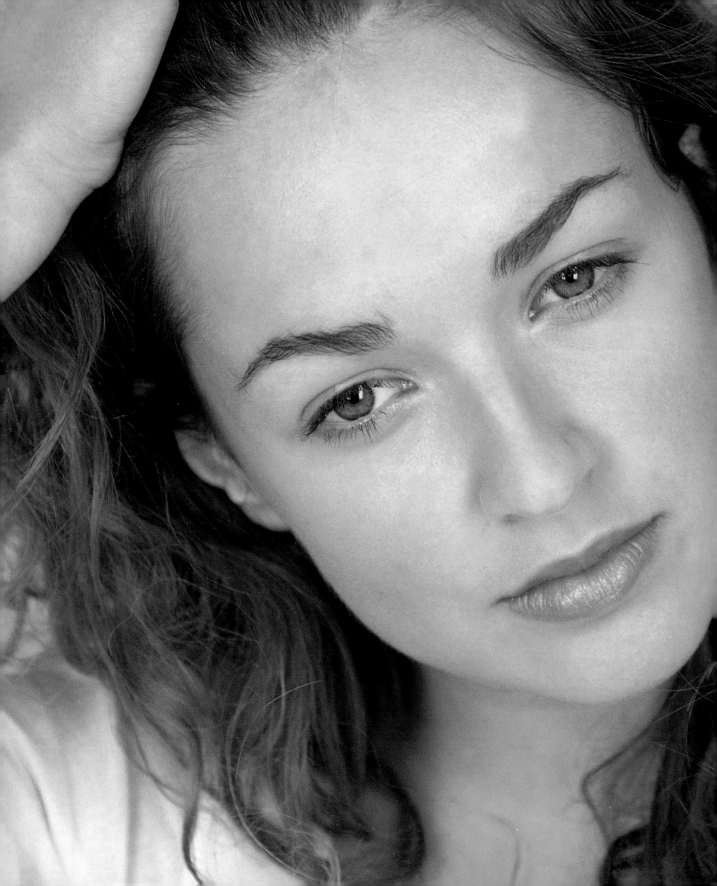

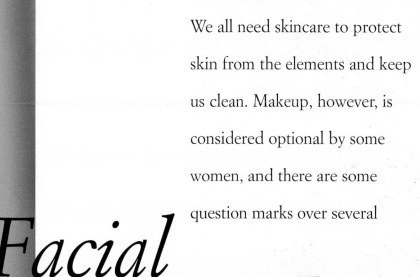

We all need skincare to protect skin from the elements and keep us clean. Makeup, however, is considered optional by some women, and there are some question marks over several

Facial beauty

makeup ingredients, particularly in lipsticks. But even wearing a small amount of makeup can have a mood-boosting impact. Read on, then, to discover the art of truly natural makeup, which not only makes you look just like you (only better), but really is as pure as nature intended.

organic *makeup*

When it comes to buying makeup, would-be organic beauties can now take a shortcut to truly natural lines that use mineral pigments in their cosmetics in place of synthetic chemicals.

We all want to look like natural beauties. In a perfect world, we could face anyone bare-faced and confident, but most of us feel we need a little extra cosmetic help. The good news is that this isn't just frivolous. Studies have shown that when women apply makeup, there's a perceptible boost to their immune system. So makeup not only makes us look good, it makes us feel better and may improve our ability to withstand infections.

NATURAL-LOOKING MAKEUP

Makeup is one area where many people compromise, prioritizing performance over natural ingredients. Not long ago, truly "natural" cosmetics meant a real tradeoff: clumpier mascara and foundation whose blendability couldn't rival those of the mainstream manufacturers in their million-dollar labs. Today, however, there are some natural lines that deliver impressive results.

Why should we worry? Our faces, after all, cover a small skin area compared with our bodies, so is a little makeup really going to hurt? Maybe. Maybe not. The jury's still out. Things have certainly improved since the time of Queen Elizabeth I, when her characteristic white makeup gave her lead poisoning, but some FD&C dyes, used in such products as eyeshadow and blusher, are a concern.

COLOR PIGMENTS

When the letters FD&C precede a color on an ingredient list, it means that the color has been approved by the U.S. Food & Drug Administration for use in foods, drugs, and cosmetics. FD&C dyes, however, are derived from coal tar; this, in turn, is derived from bituminous coal, which contains substances including benzene, napthalene, and creosol. The main concern about coal tar derivatives is that they may cause cancer. They are

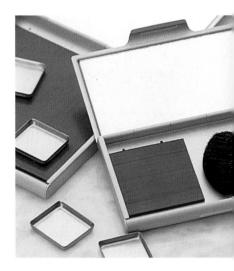

also frequently sources of allergic reactions, such as skin rashes and a prickly, heatlike effect.

Aluminum is another ingredient that worries some health-conscious consumers, because of its possible link with Alzheimer's disease. In the process of dusting on powder or blusher, we breathe in particles.

Talc comes from the same mineral group as potentially carcinogenic

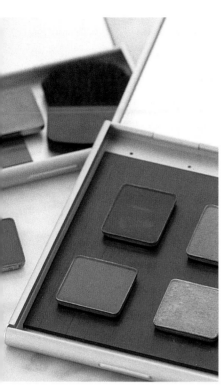

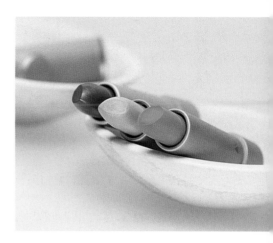

asbestos and should be avoided. In addition, many makeup lines contain mineral oil and petrolatum-derived ingredients, which are not only nonsustainable, but can also cause skin problems (see pages 10-11.)

MINERAL COLOR PIGMENTS

But there is good news. Responding to demands for truly natural makeup, not just skincare, manufacturers are starting to offer alternatives, many using mineral pigments instead of synthetic dyes and chemicals. These minerals are micropulverized, so they shield and protect the skin without making you look like you're wearing makeup.

Look for Bare Escentuals i.d. Collection and La Bella Donna Naturale Therapy makeup, which

contain nothing but pure minerals. By using ultramodern manufacturing techniques, all of these products avoid perfumes, preservatives, and oils.

Aveda (owned by Estée Lauder) have made great strides toward naturalness, with their stated policy of avoiding petrochemicals and turning to dyes such as uruku, from a South American nut, to tint their lipsticks. From a packaging point of view, Aveda also scores well, with recycled metal containers into which your color choices can be slotted.

Aveda is perhaps the most widely available choice, but many of the natural cosmetic companies offer mail order (see *Directory*, pages 122-124). Origins, the other natural arm of the Estée Lauder empire, also pledges to avoid petrochemical ingredients. Origins falls into the "trying hard" category, a medium-natural choice. The Body Shop's Colorings line, meanwhile has a policy of avoiding aluminum ingredients.

Dr. Hauschka now makes a wonderful truly natural line that avoids all potentially harmful ingredients and yet delivers amazing results. The Logona brand from Germany is equally pure; the company carries out independent laboratory tests to make sure the talc used in their products is asbestos-free.

Jane Iredale's makeup is based entirely on natural ingredients and mineral powders (zinc oxide, iron oxide, and micronized titanium dioxide), avoiding FD&C dyes,

preservatives, and fragrances. It is so nonirritating that it is prescribed by cosmetic surgeons for camouflage after facial surgery; it also offers high-level sun protection.

These guidelines apply not only to women interested in a more natural way of beauty, but also to the sensitive-skinned, too. Cut down on the number of dyes, preservatives, and fragrances in a product, and you reduce the potential for irritation.

When it comes to makeup, less really can be more, and if you use the right technique, you'll find you need less of it than you think you do.

RAINBOW WORRIES?

On cosmetic counters, you'll often find rich, high-fashion shades. Natural mineral shadows are available in some richer shades, but they tend to be mainly earth tones, which give a more natural look. If you choose rainbow-toned makeup, it's more likely to have been formulated with synthetic dye than mineral pigments. Bear that in mind when you're organic-beauty shopping.

foundation
secrets

Until now, natural foundation has meant foundation that looks natural on the skin. But you may want to start scanning labels and screening out some less-than-ecofriendly ingredients.

Fact: great-looking skin doesn't need as much camouflage as skin that is out of condition. Follow the advice given on diet and exercise, and your skin should glow and gleam, reducing the need to conceal it with foundation.

A STRONG BASE

If you are going to prioritize organic beauty choices, foundation should be high on the list. It sits on the skin, covers most of the face, and we use more of it than most makeup items. Start to scan ingredient lists and avoid foundations that contain mineral oil (*paraffinum liquidum*) and petrolatum, because they tend to block pores. That may make you more prone to lumpy red spots or to little white pimples that break out under the skin's surface. As a shortcut, without having to read the entire ingredient list, look for the expression "non-comedogenic" on the packaging; this means that the product does not block pores.

If practical (and if you like the shades offered), you would be advised to fill your makeup kit with the brands listed on pages 46-47.

You probably need less foundation than you think you do. Scrutinize your face in a mirror, although not a magnifying mirror, because that always makes everything look worse than it is. Dab foundation onto imperfections such as spots, broken veins, and dark circles, and blend well. For more coverage, use a concealer that matches your skintone perfectly. Kevyn Aucoin, one of the world's leading makeup artists, recommends the judicious use of concealer, carefully blended into the skin, in place of foundation – especially on more mature skins. Forget sponges. They're fussy, and you usually end up applying more than you need.

Foundation and concealer need setting with powder if they're not to disappear into thin air. Apply with a velvet puff pad or a brush – not the big, fluffy brush that you're usually recommended to use, but a three-quarter-inch brush that allows for precision placement of powder. Powder is normally needed only

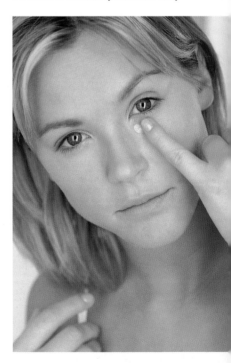

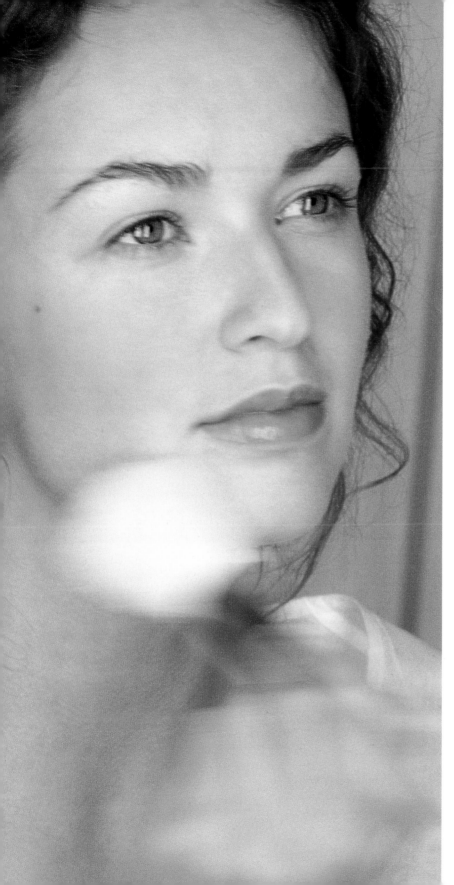

around the oily T-zone of the face: the forehead, nose, and chin.

To avoid breathing in the powder and getting a dusty effect, whack the base of the brush (or the velvet puff) hard on a flat surface before you apply it to the face.

ELIMINATING SHINE

The reason women reapply powder frequently during the day is usually to avoid shine. Oily-skinned women who follow the skincare advice on pages 26-27 should find that they start to shine less, anyway. But instead of adding powder to mop up oil, try using the one-layer-of-tissue trick on page 25. It will blot shine without disturbing the rest of your makeup.

For a sun-kissed glow, most of the companies mentioned in this makeup section make bronzing powders. For these, you should use a big, fluffy brush, the bigger and fluffier the better, and dust the bronzing powder onto your forehead, the tip of your nose, your chin, and the top of your cheekbones – anywhere the sun strikes naturally. Once you have loaded the color onto the brush, tap the handle sharply on a flat, hard surface to remove any excess, which will mean you don't apply too much to the face and that there aren't loose particles of bronzer in the air for you to breathe in.

Allow ten minutes after applying moisturizer before making up. This will encourage the makeup to stay put for longer, avoiding the need for touchups during the day.

blusher
and bronzing

A healthy glow is something we all want to achieve, especially in the depths of a gloomy winter. For the best results, buy one of the natural products mentioned here – or make your own.

The best way to get a healthy, just-got-back-from-a-brisk-walk glow is, of course, to go for a brisk walk, but blusher was invented for times when you want to be able to fake that healthy look.

The most natural blusher choices you can buy in stores come from the companies mentioned at the beginning of the makeup section: Dr. Hauschka, Logona, Jane Iredale, Aveda, Origins, and Colorings at The Body Shop. Most of these companies offer powder blushers, although Origins offers one in a gel form, much-loved by celebrities, called Pinch Your Cheeks. Just the merest dab goes a long, long way, giving a see-through flush that is ultrarealistic (provided you're not too heavy-handed.)

Many hip beauty companies offer "cheek tints" instead of cream or powder blushers, which give a natural, translucent, healthy glow. It is also incredibly easy to make your own with beet juice as described opposite.

So, once you've bought it, how should you apply it? Contrary to popular myth, the most natural-looking place for blusher definitely is not in a stripe along the cheekbone. Nobody blushes there, in real life. For a natural, flattering flush, apply blusher to the "apples" of the cheeks. Locate yours by smiling: the apple of your cheeks will bulge slightly. Apply blusher there, and blend outward using a very light touch. Use this technique, whatever formulation of blusher you choose.

CHEEK TINT RECIPE

To get that rosy-cheeked look, you can make a cheek tint at home using organic beet that gives exactly the same result as those created by some large cosmetic companies and which is, of course, 100 percent free of preservatives and artificial dyes.

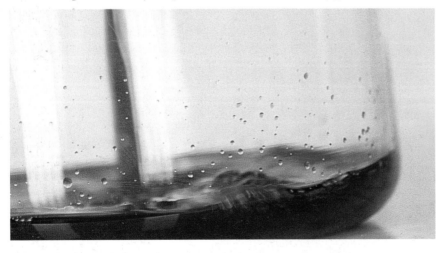

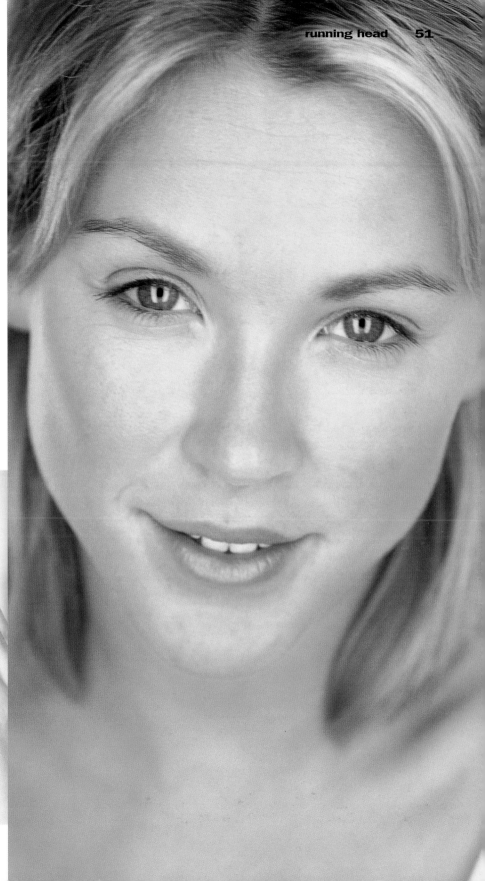

Its transparency makes it perfect for giving a natural-looking glow to bare skin for outdoor activities, but it can also be applied over foundation. Unlike powder blushers, which sit on the skin, this blusher never looks dusty. To make the cheek tint you will need:

1 tsp glycerin

4-6 drops beet juice (more for a darker tint of blusher)

Grate a raw beet and strain the resulting juice. Put the juice in a saucepan and simmer to reduce it to a quarter of its original volume (watch the pan!) When cooled, add the juice to the glycerin in a small glass bottle, using a dropper, and shake well.

Because makeup technology is so complicated, this is the only blusher that is practical to make at home.

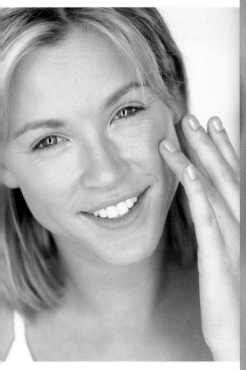

soothing
tired eyes

In our world of computers, televisions, and extended working hours, your eyes – one of your most precious features – are all too often neglected. Revive them with these refreshing recipes.

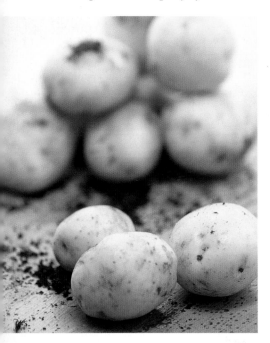

Late nights, computer work, and even reading can all take a toll on our eyes. Lack of sleep results in red-eye and dark circles. Food sensitivities, allergies to pollen, and sensitivity to some makeup can lead to puffy eyes.

The best way to put the sparkle back in tired eyes is by getting plenty of rest, but there is no need to reach for pharmaceutical eye drops when you're simply suffering from lifestyle-related soreness or redness.

FAST FIXES FOR PUFFY EYES

Swelling that doesn't disappear rapidly once you're out of bed is commonly caused by allergies, so you may need to consider whether there is anything you are reacting to, particularly if you have a tendency to allergies. Possible triggers include cosmetics, anything applied to the eye area last thing at night, or even skin mites in your mattress and bedding.

In rare cases, major swelling around the eyes can indicate more general health problems, such as circulatory disorders. If the puffiness is very noticeable or has been persistent for a long time, consult your physician.

TO SOOTHE DRY EYES

Often eyes become tired and itchy because the air is too dry. An electric humidifier can create a more eye-friendly environment, or fill your office and home with plants, and spray-mist them frequently.

TO SOOTHE TIRED EYES

Cucumber slices, raw potato slices, and witch hazel-soaked cotton pads are all extremely soothing. Eyebright is nature's sparkle-restoring herb: add 30 drops of tincture of eyebright to a glass of cool, boiled pure water, and keep it in the refrigerator; organic cotton pads soaked in it are tremendously eye-calming. Apply morning and evening.

TO TONE DOWN RED EYES

To draw attention away from red eyes, wear less makeup. Avoid eye makeup with even a hint of red, such as purple, burgundy, and pink shades.

TO REDUCE PUFFINESS

• Pour boiling water over two organic chamomile tea bags. Let the tea bags cool and then chill them in the refrigerator and, when ready to use, squeeze out the excess water, lie down, and place them over the eyes. Relax for at least 15 minutes.

• Tannins in regular tea have an anti-inflammatory effect. Follow the method above, using black or orange pekoe tea.

• Tapping the orbital bone around the eye sharply with the middle finger, moving along the bone to circle the eye, can help drain the fluid from the area, which causes puffiness.

• Make yourself an eye-rest pillow, filled with raw seeds or rice, which you can lay on the eye area. This is wonderfully restful, and the weight of the pillow helps drain fluid from the eyelids. To make the eye-rest pillow: cut two pieces of pure silk or 100-percent natural satin, approximately 5 x 9 in (12.5 x 22.5 cm), and sew, wrong sides together, to make an envelope. Leave a 1 in- (2.5 cm) gap in the side, room enough for a funnel, and pour in one cup of flax seeds or raw rice. If you like, add crushed rose petals or lavender to scent the pillow, or dried hops to help induce sleep. Handstitch the opening in the fabric to close it up.

• Stainless steel teaspoons that have been chilled in the freezer and then are pressed on the eyelids for a few minutes also work effectively at reducing puffy eyelids.

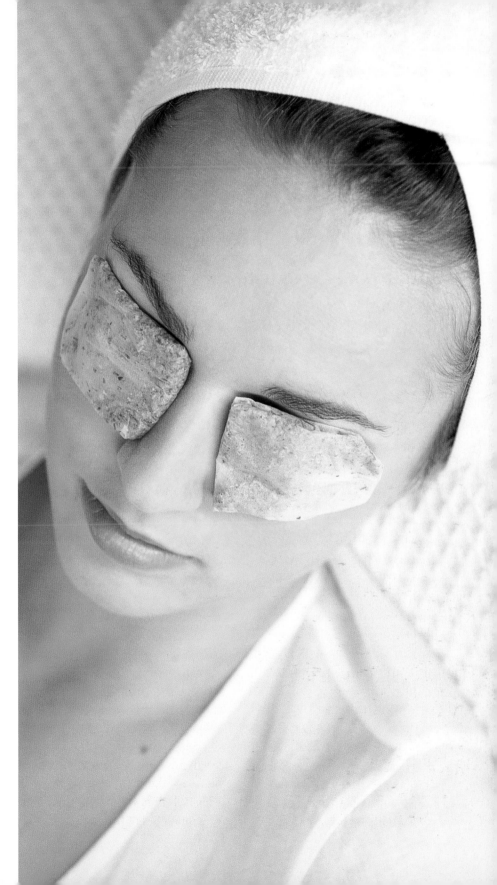

makeup
for eyes

Eyes are often the first feature you notice when meeting someone new. Make the most of your own eyes by paying them
careful attention and creating perfect – and natural – makeup.

Eyes are the windows to our souls. Long before the time of Cleopatra, women began accentuating their eyes with smoky liners. Today, mascara is the most often-quoted desert-island beauty essential, which women wouldn't want to be stranded without.

The issues for eye makeup are similar to those for other makeup: do you want mineral oil, petrolatum, chemical colorings, or aluminum in your eye makeup? If not, the cosmetic companies already mentioned make excellent alternatives that come straight from nature, not from a laboratory.

EYE MAKEUP TIPS

A light touch of foundation to eyelids helps create a smooth canvas and helps "fix" eye-shadow. The simple rule is if you're wearing more than one color of eyeshadow, place the lightest color on the brow area, the medium shade on

the eyelid, and outline the eyes (close to the lashes) in the darkest shade. You do not need "lash-lengthening" mascaras. According to makeup professionals, what really creates the illusion of long lashes is working the mascara well into the roots of the lashes. Likewise, liner can be worked into the lash-line.

Accentuate brows and lashes, and you may find you can get away with much less eye makeup than before (this is especially true for blue-eyed blondes, whose eyes can "disappear" without some color.) According to makeup artist Mary Greenwell, "eyebrows really do frame the face, drawing attention to the eyes, making them appear larger and more defined."

SHOULD EYELASHES BE DYED?

As anyone who's had their lashes dyed will tell you, it can sting and leave your eyes watering, and beauticians must

take great precautions to prevent the dye from going in the client's eyes. There may also be other health concerns about dyes (see pages 84-85.) Besides, when a mascara is as good as Dr. Hauschka's rose-scented version (which is also perfect for sensitive eyes), who needs eyelash dyes?

BRUSH NOTES

Most makeup brushes are made from animal hair and are a byproduct of the fur industry. However, Origins makes a set of "can't-tell-them-from-real-hair" brushes that do the job incredibly well. Aveda's brushes, meanwhile, are real animal hair reportedly from "humanely combed and groomed animals." The Body Shop offers a couple of synthetic brushes, as does Shu Uemura. Ask before you buy, because they are so realistic that it is difficult to tell them from those brushes made from sable, squirrel, or pony hair.

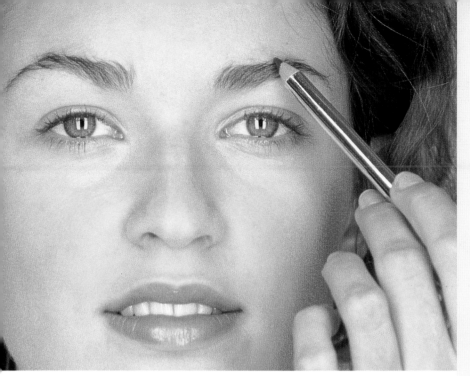

BROW KNOW-HOW

When defining your eyebrows, do so before applying the rest of your eye makeup, to frame your eyes. Use a well-sharpened pencil and light, feathery strokes, following the brow line; aim to color the brow hairs, not the skin. With a steady hand, following the brow's natural arc, you can extend the line of the brow very slightly in the direction of the ear – in this case, drawing lightly on skin. Press the line with your finger to soften, but do not smudge it.

Alternatively, use eyeshadow powder just slightly darker than your brow color and using light, feathery strokes, color the brow hairs, not the skin, following the brow's natural line. You can buy specially angled brow brushes for this purpose. To make sure the color stays on longer, try layering brow products: first pencil, then powder, to "set" the brow line. Recycle an old mascara wand as a brow groomer: cleanse it thoroughly, and use it to brush the hairs into shape after coloring. Alternatively, skim the merest dab of a balm – even a lip balm – over brows, to groom them, and brush into shape with the wand. Be careful when choosing pencils or powders that there isn't even the merest whisper of red in the color.

TO PLUCK OR NOT TO PLUCK?

Shaping the eyebrows so there's a clean arc can really open up the eye area, so you need less eye makeup. It's a question of personal preference. Just remember – unless they're plucked repeatedly, eyebrows grow back.

Before you reach for the tweezers, you might want to reflect on an ancient Mayan belief: that we actually have far more than five senses, and that brow hairs serve as extra "sensors" just like a cat's whiskers.

How to pluck eyebrows

1 Sit in natural daylight and use a handheld magnifying mirror. Cleanse the area thoroughly with a natural cleanser, and remove any last trace of the cleansing product with rosewater or witch hazel to make sure that the surface isn't greasy.

2 Using a brow pencil, draw in the brow's natural line (as explained, left) to act as a guide and prevent over-plucking. Gently pull the skin of the outer edge of your eyebrow up and out so you can see the brow bone, and use it as a guide. (Remember: brows should extend a bit farther than each corner of your eyes, so don't pluck too much from either end).

3 Pluck stray hairs first, using a sharp pair of tweezers with fine points. Makeup artists favor Tweezerman's (see *Directory,* pages 122-124).

4 Start in the middle of the brow and work toward your ear, then work from the middle in toward your nose – making sure the arch is highest at the center of the brow.

5 Always tweeze from underneath the brow, never the top, following the natural shape and plucking hair out in the direction in which it grows.

6 Wipe the area with a cotton swab dipped in pure Tea Tree Oil – nature's perfect antiseptic.

essential
lip therapy

When it comes to beauty regimes, lips are low in the pecking order. The following lipcare treatments show how to combat the drying effects of wind, central heating, and sun.

Are you addicted to lip balm? Millions of us are. Lips are protected by the thinnest skin on the body, which makes them very sensitive to touch – and one of the key erogenous zones. Since lips do not have the sweat- or oil-secreting glands that other areas of skin contain, they tend to dry out very quickly. Moistening the lips with saliva merely contributes to the drying effects, as does the Saharalike environment created by central heating and air conditioning.

Regular application of lip balm helps prevent this dryness, which can lead to cracked and sore lips (leaving the skin on the lips prone to infection). Many conventional lip balms, however, are petroleum-based, and, in my opinion, this ingredient seems to enhance their addictive appeal. Interestingly, women who switch to a wax-based or a homemade lip balm do not appear to experience the same urge to reapply the lip balm again and again.

DIY LIPCARE

Making your own lip treatments is simple (see the recipes on page 57). If you do not have time to make your own, make sure you study the ingredients list on any balm you buy, and avoid those that contain petrolatum or mineral oil. Instead, look for balms featuring high levels of wax (usually beeswax or carnauba wax).

Applied on top of your choice of lipstick or lip pencil, lip balm creates a glossy, sexy finish that not only protects but also helps lips retain their natural moisture.

HERE COMES THE SUN

During the summer, or at any time when the sun is prominent and there is little cloud cover, try to wear some sort of lip protection whenever you are outdoors. Research has shown that women are between 7-10 times less likely than men to develop lip cancer, and the fact that many women wear lipstick is thought to be the reason. Lip balm – unless it's a commercial version, with an SPF15 or more – will not offer the same level of protection as colored lipstick, in which the pigments (and titanium dioxide in the formulation) help create a shield for lips. Choose from one of the listed natural brands (see pages 46-47,) and your lips will love you for it.

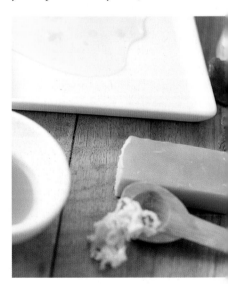

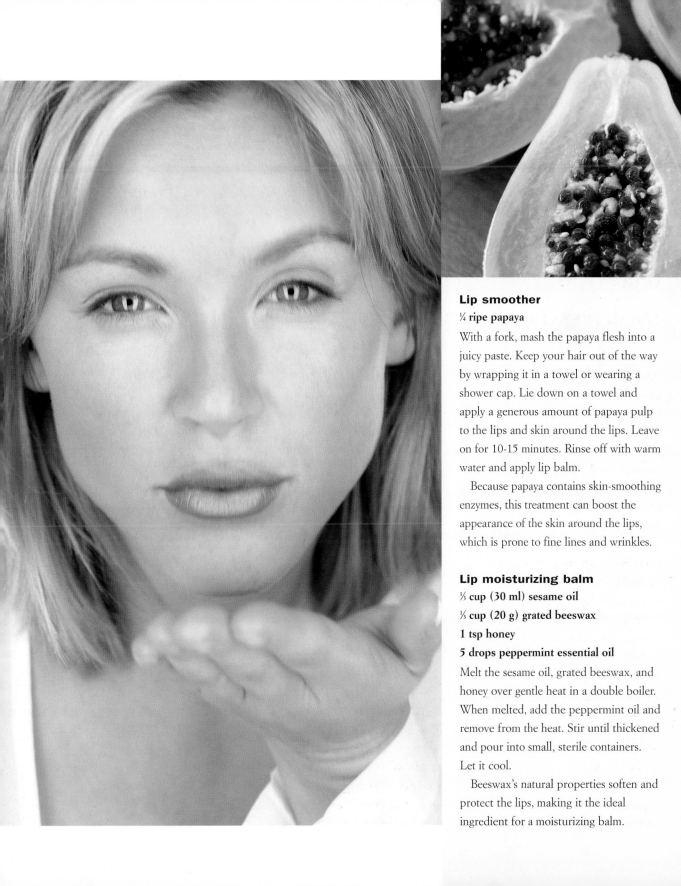

Lip smoother

¼ ripe papaya

With a fork, mash the papaya flesh into a juicy paste. Keep your hair out of the way by wrapping it in a towel or wearing a shower cap. Lie down on a towel and apply a generous amount of papaya pulp to the lips and skin around the lips. Leave on for 10-15 minutes. Rinse off with warm water and apply lip balm.

Because papaya contains skin-smoothing enzymes, this treatment can boost the appearance of the skin around the lips, which is prone to fine lines and wrinkles.

Lip moisturizing balm

⅛ cup (30 ml) sesame oil
⅛ cup (20 g) grated beeswax
1 tsp honey
5 drops peppermint essential oil

Melt the sesame oil, grated beeswax, and honey over gentle heat in a double boiler. When melted, add the peppermint oil and remove from the heat. Stir until thickened and pour into small, sterile containers. Let it cool.

Beeswax's natural properties soften and protect the lips, making it the ideal ingredient for a moisturizing balm.

natural
lip color

If you don't let nonorganic food pass your lips, it makes sense to wear only organic products on them. These pages show how to achieve perfectly made-up lips – naturally.

Lipstick has an instant feel-good factor. It is also the fastest way to update your image.

A truly natural lipstick and lip pencil should be high on your priority list because, according to Aveda founder Horst Rechelbacher, lipstick wearers consume between one-and-a-half and four tubes of lipstick in a lifetime.

We literally chew and lick lipstick and gloss off our lips, yet they often contain indigestible components such as petroleum. What's more, in order to give intense color, lipsticks may contain a very wide range of synthetic dyes and colorings, not to mention elements such as aluminum.

COLOR TO DIE FOR
In the U.S., the FDA considers many pigments potentially unsafe: only around 80 are allowed, compared with almost 200 in Europe. The natural lipsticks mentioned here use no coal tar dyes, relying on mineral pigments such as iron oxides. Some also contain a crimson food coloring called carmine, which is not suitable for vegetarians; it comes from the dried wings of a Mexican and Central American species of beetle (however the red color only exists if the beetles die a natural death, once they've mated. They're then vacuumed off the cacti they feed on and sent for extraction.)

THE NATURAL LOOK
Today, there is an increasingly wide range of 100-percent natural lipsticks on the market. Jurlique has a small collection of colors, mostly pinkish browns. Dr. Hauschka lipsticks and those from Logona (who make thick lipstick pencils) are also worth seeking out, but don't expect dramatic scarlets and deep purples, because natural pigments can't deliver that depth of color. Aveda's lipsticks, which are petrochemical-free, are tinted with organically grown uruku, a plant-derived pigment from the *Bixa orellana* plant (which grows in the Brazilian rain forest) and contain breath-freshening plant extracts, too.

Like Aveda, Origins pledges not to use petrochemical ingredients, and their line includes a lovely, glossy thick pencil lipstick, called Sheer Stick, which delivers a slick of natural-looking, shiny color.

The companies mentioned here also make lip pencils, and Logona makes a double-ended pencil sharpener out of ecologically friendly polypropylene. It has a dual blade to sharpen both thick and thin pencils.

These natural brands avoid the use of petrochemical ingredients, which are very cheap, by using natural waxes such as carnauba wax, beeswax, jojoba oil, and shea butter.

You can also make your own tinted lip gloss. Follow the recipe for the balm on page 57 and add 10 drops of beet juice to the mixture.

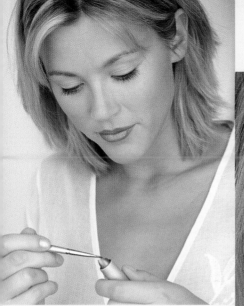

LIP TIPS

• A dab of lip balm in the center of the bottom lip creates the illusion of fuller, bee-stung lips, by catching the light.

• As an alternative to lipstick, outline the lips with a lipliner or lip pencil and literally "fill in" the outline. Apply homemade lip balm over the top for a sensuous pout. (To avoid a madeup look, blur the outline by pressing on the lip skin very lightly with your fingertip – but don't rub, or you'll smudge the outline.)

• For a longer-lasting lip tint, apply lipstick and then separate a 2-ply recycled facial tissue. Place a layer between your lips and press them together. Reapply and blot again. The pigment stays on the lips, and you're less likely to need to reapply your lipsitck during the day.

• Pencil-style lipsticks need regular sharpening with a special lip pencil sharpener or the wooden stub scratches the lips, but for a natural effect, blunt the end by drawing lightly on the back of your hand.

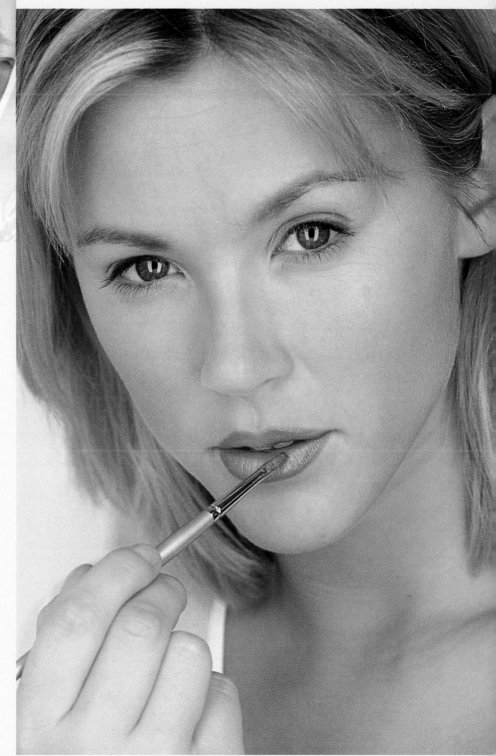

pure white
smile

With the advent of natural toothpaste and reverse-osmosis water filters, your smile and toothcare can be as healthy, natural, and chemical-free as the food you eat.

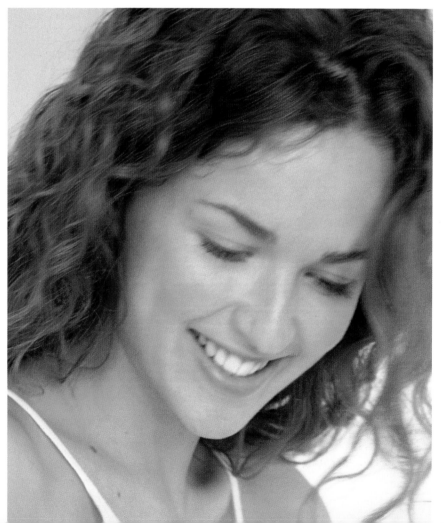

If you're choosing to go organic because you're concerned about your health, you may decide to put natural toothcare near the top of your list. Many are made of ingredients that are good enough to eat – which, if you're putting something in your mouth, makes perfect sense, since some inevitably gets swallowed.

Some parts of the body including the gums are more absorbent than others, making it easier for chemicals to pass into the bloodstream.

If someone has gum disease (with gums that bleed), that's a real short-cut for the chemicals in toothpaste to get into your system.

SMILE PLEASE

In the quest for whiter, brighter smiles, many toothpastes are a long way from pure and natural with extra chemicals such as fluoride. Many experts claim fluoride helps fight decay, yet it has also been linked, in at least eight

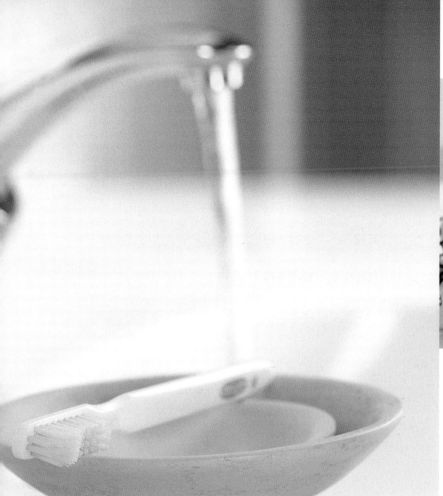

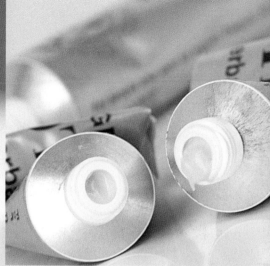

vitamins, brushing and flossing regularly, and eating calcium-rich foods such as dried peas and beans, canned fish, and dark leafy greens, including beet and turnip tops, and kale.

SOMETHING IN THE WATER

In many places, it is impossible to avoid fluoride, even by switching toothpaste, because it is actually added to the water supply by the authorities. In the long term, this may turn out to have serious health implications: there is evidence that fluoride causes dental fluorosis (resulting in white flecks on the tooth surface, or even brown mottling), and it may also be linked with a dramatic increase in hip fractures in the elderly.

There is a way around this, however: filtering your drinking water by having a reverse-osmosis water filter installed in your kitchen removes all traces of this potentially harmful chemical from your tap water.

American studies, to an increase in bone fractures. It is believed by natural health experts to interfere with the body's balance of calcium, magnesium, iron, and zinc and, in a high enough dose, it is extremely toxic.

In the U.S., toothpastes with sodium fluoride carry a "warning", and users are advised not to swallow more than the quantity required for brushing, and to keep toothpaste in a secure cabinet out of reach of children under 6.

TOOTHPASTE INGREDIENTS

Many regular toothpastes contain preservatives or foaming agents, which are given direct access to the bloodstream via the thin lining of the mouth and gums.

If you would prefer to use a natural toothpaste, look out for toothpaste by The Green People Company, Weleda, Lavera, Logona, Urtekram, and Bioforce.

THE CONVENTIONAL VIEW

You might choose to follow a conventional dentist's advice and use a mainstream fluoride toothpaste. Alternatively, go for a natural toothpaste choice, and take other positive steps to prevent cavities.

Tooth decay can be avoided by cutting out sugar, getting plenty of

oral care
recipes

Although toothpaste was one of the first organically certified beauty products, you may still like to try making your own tooth powder and mouthwash since they are so easy to create.

Try these alternatives to commercial toothpastes and mouthwashes.

BAKING SODA TOOTH POWDER

Simply dab a dampened toothbrush in baking soda, then brush your teeth. You can also add one drop of tea tree essential oil onto the brush: it serves as an antiseptic and is great if you suffer from bleeding gums.

Herbal tooth powder

This recipe is particularly good if you have fragile or bleeding gums; myrrh is a well-known treatment for gum disease, while tea tree oil works against plaque buildup.

½ cup (100 g) white clay powder

4 oz (100 g) baking soda

1 tsp dried herbs, to taste: choose from peppermint, spearmint, sage, fennel, or wintergreen

1 tsp myrrh powder

1 tsp dried raspberry leaf

1 tsp dried yellow dock root

peppermint essential oil (optional)

Pour the white clay powder and the baking soda into a mixing bowl. Grind the herbs into a powder with a spice mill or coffee grinder (or by hand in a mortar and pestle). Add all the other dry ingredients and mix well with a wire whisk. You can also add 5 drops of peppermint essential oil if you want a zingier blend. Cover the bowl with a clean towel or dishcloth and leave it overnight; in the morning, mix well again and package in an opaque, widemouthed jar. Use by wetting your toothbrush and sprinkling a little of the herb powder onto your brush; if you keep moisture out of the mixture, it will keep indefinitely.

FOR FRESH BREATH

Many people like the extra freshness of using a mouthwash after brushing or to freshen up between meals. However, some are extremely high in alcohol, and a study in 1991 of people who had used high-alcohol mouthwash at least daily for two decades, linked mouthwash use with an increased risk of cancer in the mouth and tongue zone.

If you want to use a mouthwash, look for one of the natural brands, such as Logona or Weleda. Alternatively, you can make your own with this simple non-alcoholic recipe.

Herbal mouthwash recipe

1 tbs dried eucalyptus leaves

1 tbs dried lemon balm

1 tbs dried peppermint

1 tbs dried sage

1 tbs dried rosemary

1 tbs dried thyme

Mix all the herbs together and keep in an airtight jar. Every few days, make a new batch of mouthwash by boiling 4 teaspoons of the mixture in a cup of water and letting it stand, covered, for another 10 minutes. Strain and pour into a sterilized jar with a tight-fitting lid.

Keeping the mixture in the refrigerator maintains its freshness and its ultra-refreshing taste.

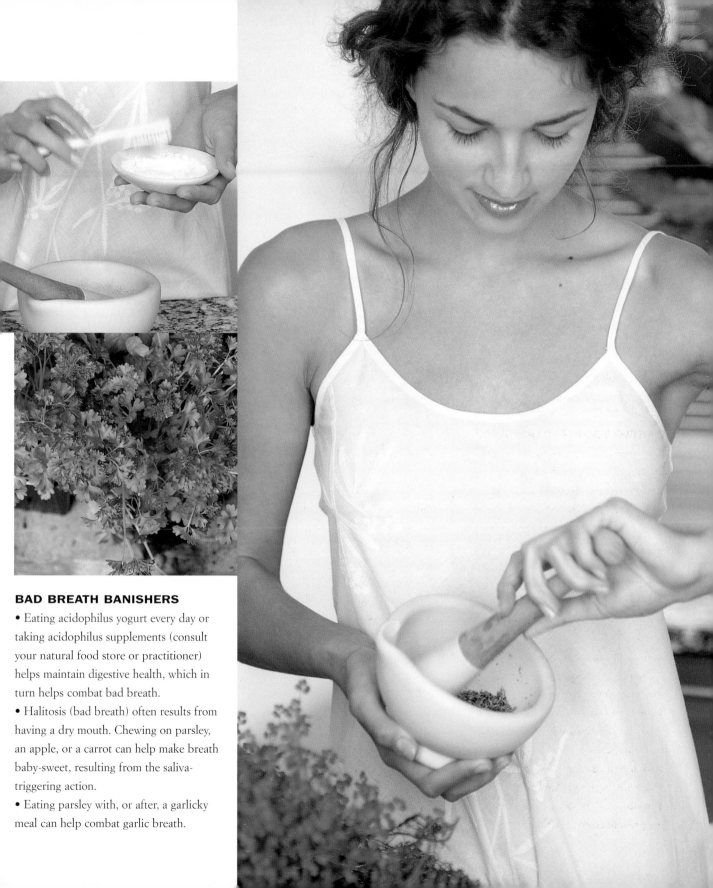

BAD BREATH BANISHERS

• Eating acidophilus yogurt every day or taking acidophilus supplements (consult your natural food store or practitioner) helps maintain digestive health, which in turn helps combat bad breath.

• Halitosis (bad breath) often results from having a dry mouth. Chewing on parsley, an apple, or a carrot can help make breath baby-sweet, resulting from the saliva-triggering action.

• Eating parsley with, or after, a garlicky meal can help combat garlic breath.

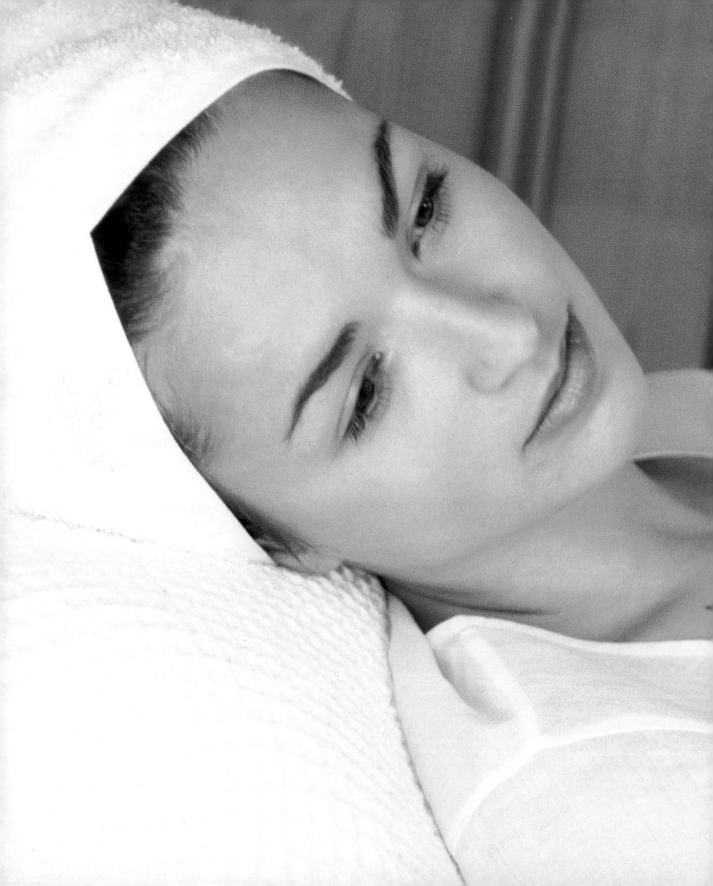

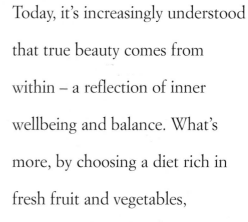

Today, it's increasingly understood that true beauty comes from within – a reflection of inner wellbeing and balance. What's more, by choosing a diet rich in fresh fruit and vegetables,

Inner beauty

drinking plenty of water and juices, and taking regular exercise, you will glow with good health from within. The key for organic beauties, of course, is to make sure that what goes into your body – feeding your whole being, not just the visible skin – is as natural and pure as possible.

eating
for healthy skin

Here are the delicious, complexion-boosting foods that should be on the menu for every organic beauty, helping to deliver healthy, vibrant-looking skin for a lifetime.

Creams, conditioners, and lotions can all help in the quest for soft skin, shiny hair, and smooth pink fingernails, but organic beauty needs a two-way approach, with diet playing an important role, too. Skin, hair, and nails all contain proteins – including elastin, keratin, and collagen – which respond to nutrients. Vitamin A, vitamin B6, and zinc must be included in the diet for healthy skin texture, strength, and moisturization. Although "fat" has (wrongly) become the enemy of many weight-conscious women, essential fatty acids (EFAs) support the body oils that keep the skin and scalp in good condition.

TO KEEP SKIN SMOOTH

Skincare companies are increasingly incorporating antioxidant ingredients in their products to help mop up the free-radical damage caused by exposure to pollution and UV light. But you can also slow this process and help shield skin from harm by upping the free-radical-scavenging antioxidants in your diet, such as vitamins C and E, and beta-carotene (which is converted in the body into vitamin A). Find vitamin C in citrus fruits, rose hips, red and green bell peppers, broccoli, and beansprouts. Vitamin E can be found in cold-pressed wheatgerm oil and cold-pressed safflower oil (which can both be added to "skin juices," see pages 68-69 for recipes). For beta-carotene, look for yellow and orange fruits and vegetables, dark leafy vegetables, and, if you're not vegetarian, liver and fish oils (be aware that high levels of pesticides, drugs, and pollutants have been found in the livers of nonorganic animals and fish.)

Zinc and selenium also seem to fight sun damage to the skin. Zinc helps with wound-healing and supports the tissue-rebuilding actions of vitamin A. Sources of zinc include seafood, egg yolk, nuts, legumes, and grains. Dr. Karen Burke, a renowned New York dermatologist, has found in research on animals that selenium greatly reduces the incidence of ultraviolet-induced skin cancer – although this research has yet to be translated to humans. Selenium also helps with vitamin E absorption.

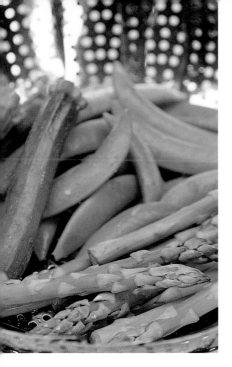

ESSENTIAL FATTY ACIDS

Many people resist fats of all types, but your body and skin need some fat to operate healthily. Experts suggest increasing the intake of essentials fatty acids (EFAs), such as omega-3s and omega-6s, since they lubricate from the inside. Skin all but shouts for this essential nutrient: dry, flaky skin and hair and cracking nails are common signs of EFA deficiency. The trick is to consume beneficial fats and minimize harmful fats. Flax seeds, linseeds, and oily fish are high in EFAs. High on the banned list should be hydrogenated fat, found in a range of mainstream foods. It is not permitted in organic food, so you automatically cut out this ingredient – thought to interfere with healthy fat metabolism – if you eat organic.

Getting the right balance of omega-3s and omega-6s is complicated, but there are premixed blends on the market, such as Udo's Choice Maximum Nutrition and Spectrum Oils Essential Max (see *Directory*, pages 122-124). Ask in your natural food store for others. Alternatively, start sprinkling flax seeds generously on your food. Every day (the mixture needs to be kept very fresh), place one to two tablespoons of flax seed into your herb mill or blender and whizz them into flax meal. Throughout the day, sprinkle a generous portion on all types of food – cereals, sandwiches, stews, casseroles.

If you eat well, it isn't hard to get the optimum dose of these skin vitamins and nutrients, but if you'd like to supplement your diet with vitamin pills and capsules, most natural food stores have an in-house expert. Don't "self-medicate" with vitamins; in excess, some are harmful. Try, wherever you can, to get as many vitamins as you can from food.

To keep your digestive system in good order, eat at least an ounce of fiber daily and, to eliminate toxins, hydrate skin, and flush out your system, drink plenty of water (see pages 72-73).

TO CLEAR UP PROBLEMS

Acne responds to a wide range of nutrients. Vitamin A, for instance, has been found by some doctors to clear it up, partly because it helps reduce the production of pore-clogging sebum. If you feel you need to take a supplement, you could try – after consultation with your doctor or a natural health professional – taking vitamin A supplement daily. Women who are pregnant, however, or trying to conceive should *not* take high doses of vitamin A, because it is linked with an increased risk of birth defects.

Low levels of zinc have been observed in some acne sufferers, so try increasing your intake. EFAs also seem helpful at relieving inflamed skin, because they increase the skin's resilience and "good" lubrication.

Vitamin B6 may be helpful for PMS-related flare-ups, because it helps to balance hormone levels. It can be found in oily fish, yogurt, eggs, legumes, peanuts, bananas, avocados, cauliflower, and liver. Whenever possible, try to get these nutrients from foods.

THE BASIC RULE

Eat a balanced, varied, organic diet that incorporates plenty of fresh fruit, vegetables, and whole grains. If you're not vegetarian, boost your intake of oily fish and shellfish and eat brown rice, bananas, yogurt, potatoes in the skin, pumpkin seeds, sea vegetables, green leafy vegetables, fresh fruit, sauerkraut, apples, and sheep's milk products.

Throw a handful of seeds into cereals, salads, and stir-frys. Your skin will love you for it.

juicing
for good health

Here's the fastest, easiest way to make sure you get your recommended five servings of fruit and vegetables a day. Fresh fruit and raw vegetable juices are nature's best rejuvenators.

The simplest way to get a dose of skin-boosting nutrients is with juicing. Some experts in longevity believe that the path to agelessness, not to mention maximum life span, is through the consumption of "live" foods and the supplementation of raw vegetables and fruit juices. Juicing fans also swear that fasting this way swiftly purifies the body, ridding it of potentially harmful buildup of toxins (such as agrochemicals and other pollutants, which may linger in the digestive system).

A HEALTHY SNACK

Juices are an easy and delicious way to make sure we are getting our quota of fruit and vegetables each day, which can be hard to achieve otherwise. Few of us would eat five carrots, but we could easily drink a 16-ounce glass of carrot juice, which is the equivalent. Taken with meals, the enzymes in fresh juice help us digest our foods. Juices are also great meal substitutes when

you are in a hurry and need a fast blast of nutrients.

JUICING SECRETS

Invest in a juicing machine if you're going to drink juices on a regular basis. No two juices need be the same – the only limit is your imagination. Make sure you drink a combination

of fruit and vegetable juices to get the maximum nutritional benefit. It goes without saying that if you're juicing, you should stick exclusively to organic ingredients. Berries, for example, may have been sprayed many times over, so if you juice nonorganic fruit and vegetables, you're juicing pesticides, too.

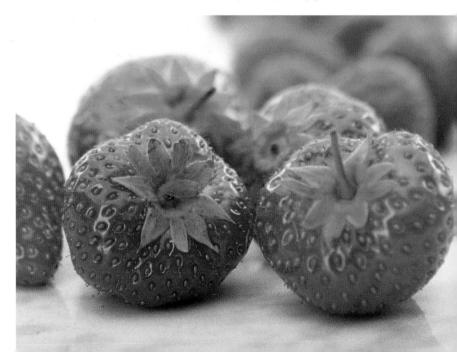

• Look upon each glass of juice as a meal in itself. Sip slowly – that way, the enzymes present in your saliva start to break it down even before the juice reaches the stomach.

• To begin with, start with up to three 8-ounce glasses of juice a day – veterans can up the amount to six glasses. (Because fruit juice causes a rapid rise in blood sugar, anyone suffering from candidiasis, low blood sugar, or diabetes should take professional advice before upping their intake of fresh juices).

• Drink the juice as soon as possible after making; fresh juices quickly lose their vitamin content.

• Great skin-boosting ingredients include carrots, orange and yellow fruit and vegetables, and leafy green vegetables (providing beta-carotene and vitamin A). Acne and dry, rough skin will particularly respond to juices with these ingredients.

• Flavonoids are essential for holding our tissues together. They're particularly rich in blueberries, blackberries, cherries, grapes, and fruit skin. The white part of the inner rind of grapefruit, oranges, and bell peppers will help strengthen capillary walls, so try incorporating these in juices if you suffer from broken veins or bruise easily.

• Potassium is an important mineral for skin elasticity and can be found in sea vegetables (such as dulse), bananas, carrots, parsley, kale, kelp, and spinach. The skin also thrives on organic sulfur – as found in fresh garlic.

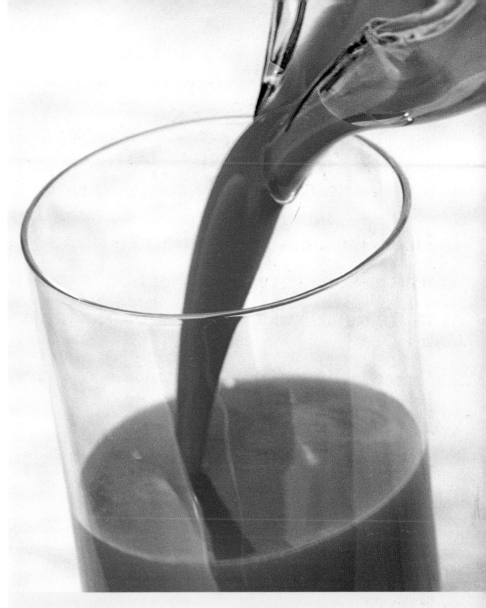

Megaskin juice
1 red bell pepper
1 green bell pepper
1 medium cucumber
Juice each ingredient, then blend together using a spoon. To keep skin clear of blemishes, well-toned, and healthy, you need juices that are high in vitamins C and E, and beta-carotene and the minerals zinc and potassium, which stimulate the digestive system and kidneys to work efficiently.

Green face-saver
3 apples
1 handful of spinach
Wash the spinach, juice each ingredient, then blend. This combination cleanses the digestive tract and improves elimination of waste, giving your complexion a glowing boost. Drink twice a day, especially before bedtime, for maximum impact. For extra energy, you can also add a capsule of blue-green algae to the mix.

exercising
for flawless skin

When it comes to skincare, what you put in and on your body are not the only considerations. Keeping yourself supple and toned is just as important for a healthy, glowing appearance.

Skin needs to breathe. Seven percent of the oxygen you take into your lungs is used directly by the skin. Breathing in supplies cells with essential oxygen, while breathing out removes waste, including carbon dioxide (which would poison your cells if left for long enough). If we don't breathe properly, we feel less than well, and not only our skin but every part of our bodies ages more quickly.

In the high-tech, marble beauty-hall world, "oxygen" is a buzzword: it's being incorporated into skin creams and body lotions, or facials that mist pure oxygen onto the skin. But there's a better way to deliver oxygen to the complexion – exercise.

HOW EXERCISE WORKS

When you work out, oxygen rushes to every cell in your body, encouraging the whole circulatory and nervous system to perform more efficiently. Researchers at the University of Wisconsin have also established that the more oxygen you take in, the less likely you are to suffer free-radical damage, which is linked to premature aging of the skin.

The key is to get the lungs and heart working, with aerobic exercise: brisk jogging and walking, running, cycling, dynamic yoga, rebounding (on a mini-trampoline), mountain hiking, ball games (tennis, badminton, volleyball, basketball), spinning (on special bikes at gyms), rollerblading, skiing, skipping, swimming, or dancing. By making your heart work harder, exercise also raises the skin temperature, turbo-charging oxygen supplies to the skin, and allowing cells to regenerate faster and nutrients to be absorbed. It's a simple fact: exercise does more for your skin than any cream and can deliver many more physical benefits.

What does it take to make sure your skin and the rest of your organs are getting enough oxygen? Five 30-minute sessions a week, which sounds like a lot but isn't that hard to achieve, once you get in the habit. Briskly walking at least part of your journey to work means you're already incorporating regular exercise into your routine – and think of the transportation fares or parking fees you've saved in the process.

If you are completely unused to exercise, start with eight minutes a day every other day for the first week, then add three minutes per session each week. Before you know it, you'll be both slimmer and fitter, and your skin will positively glow with good health.

Of course, exercise does more than deliver a glow to the cheeks. Try to make sure that alongside your aerobic exercise you include weight-bearing or resistance exercises, such as swimming, to keep bones and muscles healthy. Above all, create a program that suits your lifestyle and you will keep up.

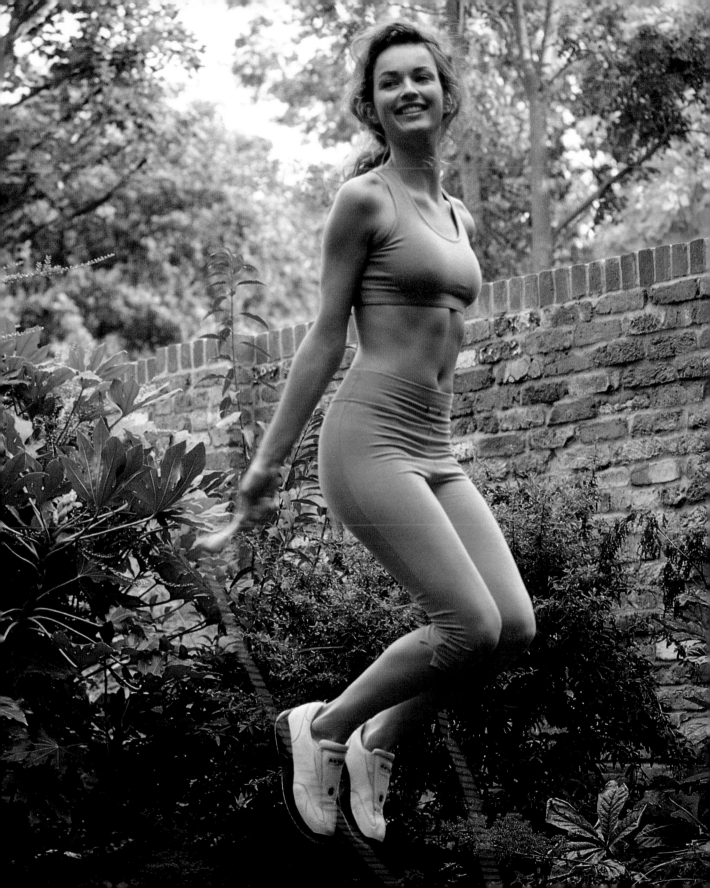

why
water works

Each of us is made up of about 63 percent water – and every supermodel you ask swears that it is her ultimate beauty secret. Here's how to make sure the water you drink is pure.

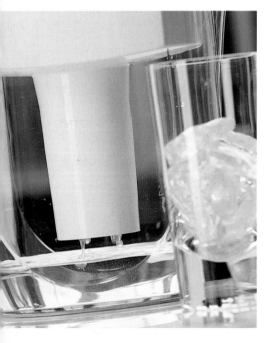

According to some skin experts, the fountain of youth may literally be found at the water drinking fountain. In our search for younger, healthier skin, drinking plenty of water is often overlooked. As if environmental stress doesn't do enough damage to the skin from the outside, stress takes its toll from the inside by dehydrating cells. You know that dry-mouth feeling you get when you're anxious about speaking in front of a room of people? That dehydration is happening in your brain and your skin, too.

TWO QUARTS A DAY

Certainly, the fastest antidote to stress is to drink a long, cool drink of water. When the skin is hydrated, the body functions more efficiently as the circulation to the skin increases.

Supermodels are always boasting that they glug a quart of water a day. According to leading nutritionist Jane Clarke, even that is not enough: we should actually be aiming for two to three quarts of water per day. Ideally, this should be either in the form of plain water or fresh organic juiced fruits and vegetables that have a high water content.

You may find it hard to achieve this level of water intake. To start with, try always keeping a glass of water on your desk, which will encourage you to remember to drink regularly. In Ayurvedic medicine, incidentally, hot water is preferred to cold, since it is easier for the body to assimilate. Personally, I feel you should drink water the way you prefer it – because then you're more likely to reach your two-to-three-quart daily target.

ATTAINING PURITY

The supply of water from your faucet may contain fluoride, arsenic, lead, and pesticides, among other harmful chemicals. To keep your drinking water pure, at the very least you should use a jug filter, which works like a coffee filter: pour the water through, and it drips into a pitcher. Alternatively, you could install a water filter on your faucet. Some have screens, or filters, that may be made from carbon or stainless steel. The

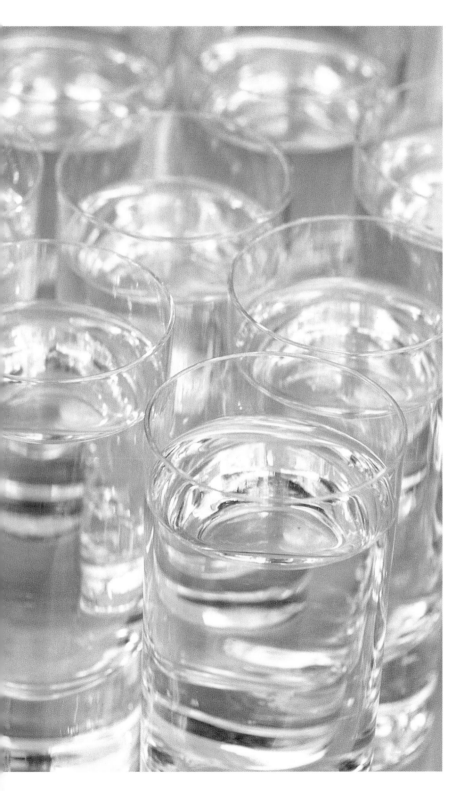

state-of-the-art system for filtering water, however, is a process called reverse osmosis: it not only filters out chemicals and pollutants but even radioactive contaminants. These filters are very expensive, but if you buy a lot of bottled water (see below), they may end up saving you money.

It is now even possible to get a whole-house unit for water filtration, rather than one that is linked to the kitchen faucet. They are designed to remove the most common contaminants, including pesticides, herbicides, and chlorine, from all the house's water. The unit is specially recommended for people with skin disorders and chemical sensitivities, but they may be beneficial to everyone – some experts claim that absorption through the skin may have been grossly underestimated (see pages 108-109). However, these filters are expensive.

If you drink bottled water, seek brands whose sources are from very deep springs. The deeper the spring, the less the chance of contamination by nuclear fallout and pesticides.

THE PROBLEM WITH CAFFEINE

People who drink a lot of tea, coffee, and cola drinks are more likely to have tired-looking skin. This is because caffeine prevents the body from making good use of the vitamins and minerals found in food.

Drink no more than two or three cups of caffeinated drinks a day, and cut out nonorganic cola drinks, since the phosphoric acid in them is linked with an increased risk of osteoporosis.

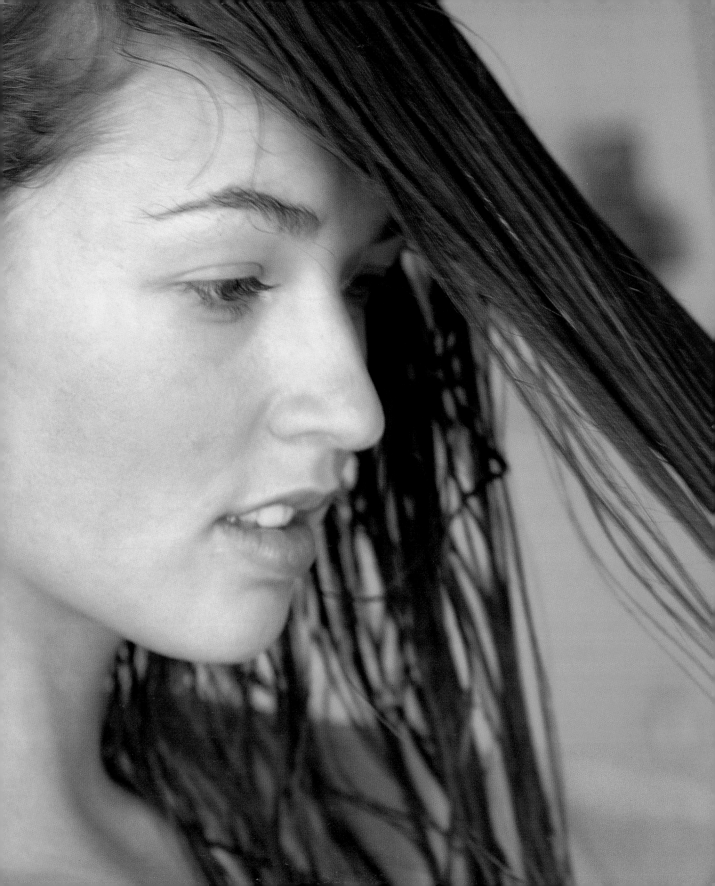

Your hair reveals much more about your health and wellbeing than just your choice of hairstyle. For many of us who live in polluted cities, haircare is a bigger priority than ever before. But did

Natural
haircare

you know that the scalp is the most absorbent part of the body, readily absorbing what you put on it? This includes shampoos, conditioners, styling products, and chemical hair colorants. Natural-as-possible haircare choices, then, should be high on the list for organic beauties.

choosing
organic haircare

"Natural" and "organic" are words that are commonly used on packaging to describe haircare products, but are virtually meaningless. Follow this guide to truly natural treatments.

Well-groomed, healthy-looking hair boosts self-confidence and our overall sense of wellbeing. Achieving that glossy, head-turning sheen through buying genuinely natural haircare should certainly be a shopping priority.

According to experts such as Ronnie McGrail, founder of Danish ultra-natural beauty company Urtekram (which is Danish for "good things,") "the scalp is the most absorbent part of the body's skin, particularly the very top (or pate)." What's more, the drying detergent action of shampoo, which interferes with the scalp's natural barrier function, makes it even easier for chemicals to penetrate. Yet increasingly, manufacturers are suggesting that shampoo be left on the scalp as a "treatment" before rinsing, and some leave-in conditioners are designed not to be rinsed off at all.

There is probably more hype about "natural" ingredients in haircare than any other area of cosmetics, some of which brazenly call themselves organic. Many are far removed from what The Soil Association in Britain would define as an organic product.

We love the idea of herbs and botanical ingredients nurturing our hair back to health, but while many mainstream herbal shampoos claim to be natural, most contain only minuscule amounts of herbs and botanical ingredients, while being loaded with preservatives and detergents.

Water and detergent make up almost all of a conventional shampoo's formulation, featuring at the beginning of ingredient labels (which must be listed in descending order), with the active elements, often adding up to no more than one percent. It is not whether the tiny amount of herbs in a product have organic certification that really matters; it is what makes up the bulk of the hair product formulation.

You might want to be aware of

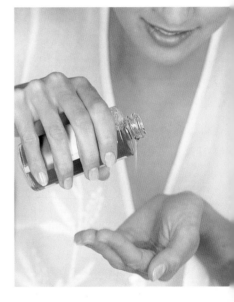

particular concerns about certain detergents; some of them feature on the list of *10 Things You Don't Want in Your Cosmetics,* on page 16. Steer clear of cocamide DEA, ammonium laureth sulfate, and sodium lauryl sulfate (SLS), which has been questioned as a cancer-causing ingredient (although a research panel organized by the

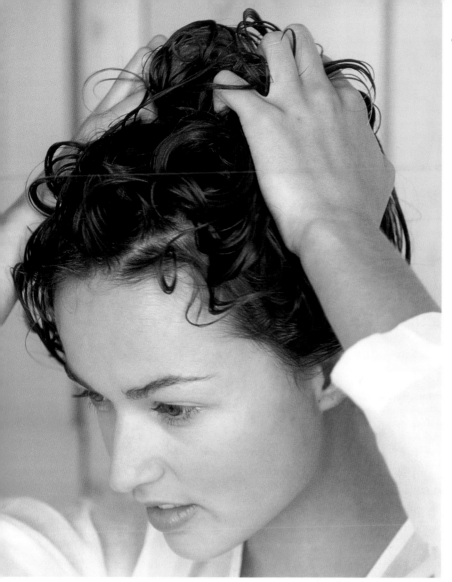

herb, which may deliver less-than-acceptable results in a world that worships squeaky clean hair.

It is more practical to use shampoo bought in a natural foodstore, such as those bought from Dr. Hauschka, Weleda, Logona, Green People, Urtekram, Aubrey Organics, Avalon Organics, Aveda, and Neways. Many of them are more concentrated than the shampoos you're used to – so a little goes a long way. Reducing the water content in shampoo means that manufacturers can use minimum (or even zero) preservatives. Aim to buy conditioner from the same brands or create your own, easy-to-blend, bliss-to-use masks, rinses, and treatment oils, suited to your hairtype, which you'll find on pages 78-83.

HAIR IN THE SUN

Hair is very vulnerable to sun, salt, and chlorine, so it needs protecting. Colored, permed, curly, and fine types are particularly porous and need even more care and attention. Go for easy-care styles, or wear your hair up or under a hat.

To protect hair against chlorine, dilute one part grapeseed oil to 15 parts water in a spray bottle. Shake to mix well and spray onto damp hair; comb out and don't rinse before going in the water. Shampoo nightly with an ultragentle shampoo to remove chlorine, sand, and salt buildup, and treat regularly with one of the nourishing masks or hair oil recipes on pages 78-83.

independent Cosmetic Ingredient Review, based in Washington, concluded that "SLS appears to be safe in formulations designed for discontinuous, brief use, followed by thorough rinsing.")

In your quest for organic haircare products, avoid highly perfumed shampoos and conditioner – the fragrance alone may contain up to 200 different chemicals and synthetic colors that have a number preceded by FD&C.

In a world where organic has become synonymous with purity and health, it is all too easy to be seduced, at first glance, by so-called "natural" haircare. Once again, reading labels is important. Buying products in a natural food store helps also, since most of their brands are striving to create truly natural products.

I would love to say that making your own shampoo is practical. It certainly can be done, but it is complicated to create an effective product at home – requiring the use of grated castile soap (which is olive-oil-based), or soapwort

problem
hair treatment

If your hair is sending out an S.O.S. – if it's greasy, oily, or it is looking rather thin and lackluster – discover these ultimate botanical hairsavers to help put back some natural bounce.

OILY HAIR

Does your hair tend to be greasy? Do you need to wash it every day? Does it rarely feel clean for more than a few hours? If so, you have oily hair.

• Give your scalp a treatment every 10 days with 4 teaspoons of jojoba oil (which helps control overactive sebaceous glands) to which you've added 20 drops of juniper oil, sage oil, or tea tree oil (or any combination of the three). Apply the oil to dry, unwashed hair, starting at the ends and moving up, always working the oil into the hair in a downward motion, to make the hair cuticle lie flat. Comb it through. To spread the oils, blow-dry your hair for approximately five minutes. For optimum results, leave the treatment on the hair for between 20 minutes and overnight. To cleanse, apply a dollop of shampoo to your palms and massage into the scalp, slowly adding water to lather up. Rinse with lukewarm water, repeat, and apply conditioner; rinse again.

• Scalp massage encourages sebaceous glands to normalize and helps prevent clogging of hair follicles.

• Wash hair daily, but use a very gentle shampoo: harsh shampoos send the sebaceous glands into overdrive. Look for shampoos with plant-based astringents such as peppermint, sage, tea tree, juniper, and lemon. Dilute one teaspoon of shampoo in one teaspoon of water to make it more gentle.

• Condition the ends of the hair only; this keeps hair healthy but stops product buildup.

• Keep your hands out of your hair. Sweaty palms make it more greasy.

• Honeydew melon works wonders on oily hair. Mash or blend a quarter of a melon, then run the juice through your hair. Leave on for 10 minutes, then shampoo and rinse out.

• Eat plenty of vitamin B2 (in eggs, brewer's yeast, whole grains, liver, and spinach), and avoid fatty, greasy foods. In particular, avoid hydrogenated fat, because it interferes with the body's own innate ability to regulate the activity of fats and oils in the body.

DANDRUFF

Do you suffer from dandruff? Does your scalp itch and flake? Once this was called dandruff. Nowadays, hairdressers prefer to call it dry scalp, which in most cases is really the cause. Dry scalp may occur more in winter, when air indoors is dry. (*Sebhorraic dermatitis* and psoriasis can also cause dandruff; if the following treatments don't work, consult your natural health practitioner or doctor.)

• Blend two tablespoons each of mineral water, olive oil, and lemon juice, then massage into the scalp. Leave for 15 minutes, shampoo, and rinse. Olive oil helps remoisturize the scalp and prevents buildup of dead skin cells; lemon juice is antibacterial and helps the skin exfoliate.

• Simple changes such as eating more oily fish and sprinkling olive oil on your salads (or using it on bread in place of butter) will greatly improve the condition of your scalp.

• Massage a cup of fresh or bottled apple juice into the hair, from roots to tips, after each shampoo. Rinse with 2 tablespoons of apple juice diluted in a quart of water.

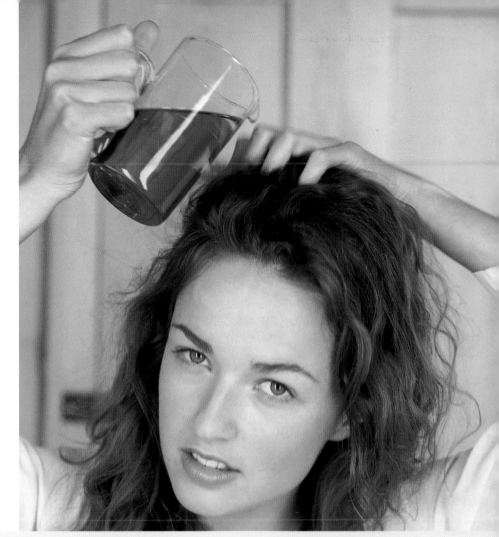

SIMPLE DANDRUFF RINSE

Say farewell to dandruff by adding a pinch each of comfrey root, rosemary, nettle, and lavender (fresh or dried) to one cup of witch hazel.

Let the herbs infuse the witch hazel for 3-5 days, when the mixture will start to smell gloriously of lavender and rosemary. Strain out the herbs, then use the liquid direct, massaged into a clean scalp (it soon dries), or as a scalp rub before bedtime.

This useful recipe also doubles as a deodorant. To use, apply it with an organic cotton pad.

Oily hair herbal rinse

1 tsp burdock root
1 tsp chamomile
1 tsp calendula flowers
1 tsp lavender flowers
1 tsp ground/chopped lemongrass
1 tsp sage leaves
1 tbs vinegar

Combine all the herbs in a large container. Pour 1 pint of boiling water over the herbs and let them steep for 30 minutes. Then strain the liquid and add 1 tablespoon of vinegar.

After shampooing, pour the liquid over your scalp and hair. Leave it on, without rinsing.

Treatment for thining hair

2 oz (50 g) avocado (or olive oil), warmed
8 drops rosemary essential oil
8 drops lavender essential oil
8 drops sage essential oil

Monthly intensive oil treatments can help all kinds of hair, but this recipe is especially suitable for boosting thinning hair or stimulating hair regrowth.

Massage into freshly washed, damp hair, then cover with a plastic shower cap or plastic wrap, and a warm towel over the top. Leave on for two hours. Rinse hair thoroughly with warm water; shampoo, and condition as normal.

dry and
colored hair

Dry and chemically treated hair needs extra-special attention to look its best. The following tips show you how to use fresh ingredients to keep your crowning glory in perfect condition.

Do you dye your hair? Do you blow-dry it every day? Is it brittle and parched, maybe even breaking easily while you're combing or brushing?

If you answered yes to any of the above, the chances are you've got dry hair. The cause may be due to blocked hair follicles that prevent the hair's natural oils from performing their moisturizing task; alternatively, the problem may stem from hair being overexposed to the sun or chemicals.

DRY HAIR

The good news is that although, strictly speaking, hair is dead, it is also porous. Think of hair as being like a sponge: apply rich conditioning ingredients, and hair becomes pliant and soft to the touch.

• Wash your hair two to three times a week, and use a mild shampoo.

• Avoid perms and straighteners, all of which are highly chemical hair treatments and savage to hair.

• Eat hair-friendly foods and supplement your diet with one to three teaspoons of flaxseed oil (it can be bought at natural food stores), a good oil that helps nourish from within.

• Vitamin E, in doses of 200 IU to 400 IU per day, can also help with dry hair, but you should always check first with a natural health nutritionist or physician before self-prescribing.

• Stay away from hairdryers, hot rollers, and curling irons, aiming instead for a low-maintenance hairstyle that doesn't require you to use them.

• Get your hair trimmed regularly. Usually, it is the ends rather than the roots that are dry; having half an inch regularly trimmed keeps the ends from getting damaged further.

• Avoid styling products that contain alcohol ingredients such as isopropyl or ethyl alcohol, both of which dry hair out even more.

• Be good to your hair by giving it regular hot oil treatments.

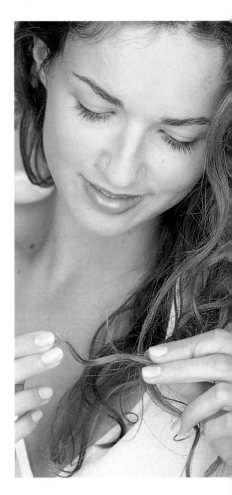

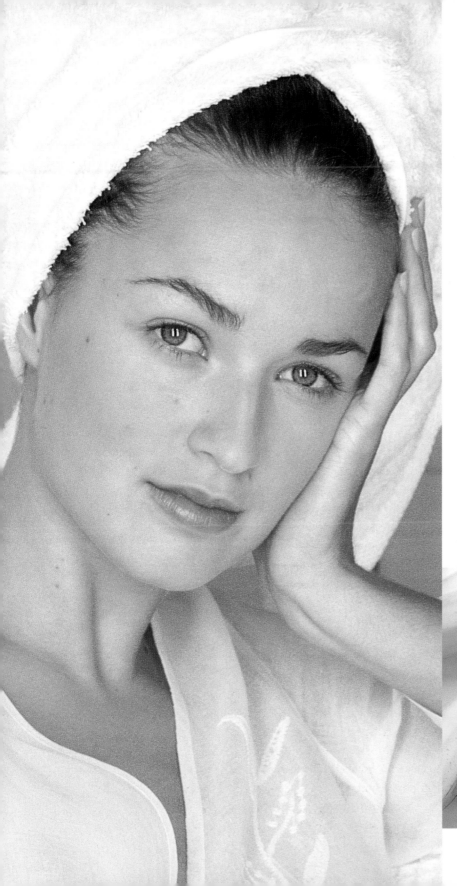

Banana hair mask

1 ripe banana

1 tbs olive oil

Mash the ingredients together and smooth onto the hair – from the roots all the way to the ends – with your hands. This procedure may be messy, but it's well worth it. Massage the mask into your hair and scalp, then wrap your hair in plastic wrap or a hot towel for 15 minutes. Rinse, shampoo, and condition as normal.

Hair mulch

1 egg white

2 tbs extra-virgin olive oil

2 tbs natural yogurt

1 tsp red wine vinegar

Beat the egg white and place in a bowl with all the other ingredients. Apply to wet hair, massage in well, and leave for 10 minutes. Because the mixture is very runny, use it while you are having a bath.

To remove, shampoo your hair twice, or until the mulch has all washed away. Condition the hair as usual.

normal
hair treatment

If you have the bonus of "normal" hair, make sure it stays that way with the following tips and ideas for making the most of one of your most important assets.

Is your hair well-behaved? Neither lank nor strawlike? No split ends? Lucky you. Your hair has the right balance of oils on the scalp, without tending toward excessive oiliness or dryness. Using the right products and techniques will help you maintain that balance.

• Shampoo only as often as your hair really needs it – which may be less often than you are in the habit of doing. Use a gentle shampoo, and dilute it with plenty of water. If it foams well the first time, you don't need a routine second shampoo.

• Use conditioner sparingly. If you find that, with the help of a wide-toothed comb and the spray attachment from your shower, you're able to detangle hair well enough without, you may not need rich conditioners or hair masks.

• Give your scalp a weekly massage. To do so, pour three drops of lavender oil onto your fingertips, rub them together to distribute it, and then massage. Refer to the "how to" instructions on pages 88-89. Massaging boosts the blood flow to the scalp and encourages healthy hair growth.

TIPS FOR EVERY HAIR TYPE

• According to experts, a final cool rinse helps close the hair cuticles (which open when exposed to hot water), resulting in greater shine.

• Air-dry your hair whenever you can. Blow-drying can damage the hair, causing split ends. If you must blow-dry, make sure that hair is really towel-dry, first. To help with this, you can now buy super-absorbent towels, such as those from Aquis, which mop up excess water. Choose a high-wattage hairdryer (1800 watts) that blasts the hair with air – rather than a slow hairdryer, to minimize drying time.

• Always remember to wear a hat in the sun. It prevents sun damage and helps keep hair from drying out. If you are going in the pool or ocean, soak hair in fresh water first so it will absorb less of the salt or chlorine. Better still, apply a mask or natural conditioner to "seal" and protect the hair cuticles before you swim.

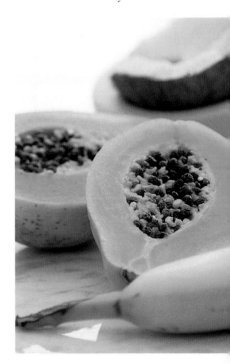

AVOCADO MASK

The natural oils in avocado make this fruit an excellent moisturizer for every hair type, except oily. Just mash the avocado, massage into the hair, cover with a shower cap, and rinse out after 30 minutes. Shampoo and condition as normal.

No-rinse conditioner

3 drops carrot-seed essential oil (if this is hard to find, substitute neroli)
3 drops chamomile essential oil
3 drops lavender essential oil
3 drops rosemary essential oil

Mix the ingredients in the palm of your hand and apply immediately (wash hands afterward.) This scalp-stimulating hair-gleamer can be applied to towel-dried hair (not scalp) after shampooing; it penetrates immediately, so there's no need to rinse.

Hair fruit salad

½ banana
1 tsp lime juice
2 tbs coconut milk
1 tbs papaya juice

Mix the ingredients well and apply to towel-dried hair. Comb through well, put on a shower cap, then wrap in a towel.

To turbo-charge the effects of the "fruit salad," aim a hairdryer at the towel to warm it (from a distance of about 1 ft.). Shampoo twice and rinse as normal.

Once you have mastered the art of using this hair salad, try experimenting with different tropical fruits – preferably fleshy rather than citrus fruits – since they will produce a thicker hair treatment. Also you could try adding advocado to the mix, which contains shine-boosting natural oils.

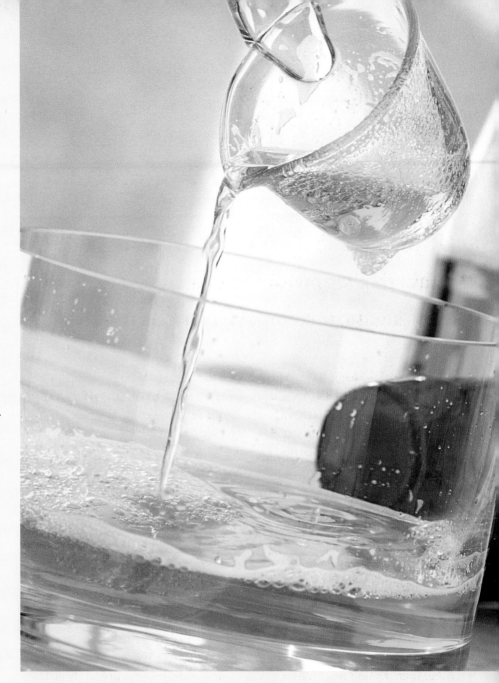

Straight-from-the-bar-rinse

2 cups (400 ml) organic ale
½ cup (100 ml) cider vinegar

Mix the organic ale and cider vinegar together in a glass measuring cup and pour over your head as a final rinse after shampooing. Let it dry naturally.

Do not be afraid to experiment with other natural ingredients to make hair rinses and treatments. As you become familiar with making your own beauty treatments from fresh fruits, vegetables, base oils, and essential oils, you'll discover what your hair type responds to best. However, if your scalp is particularly sensitive, perform a patch test first.

organic *hair color*

Nature has ways of helping us enhance our natural hair color without resorting to chemicals. Consider the increasing number of herbal hair colors available, or try making your own.

Women were coloring their hair with natural elements such as lemon, chamomile, beets, coffee, walnuts, and turmeric long before hair laboratories came up with synthetic dyes. Today, most people reach for a pack of hair dye or go to a colorist, but there have been some concerns about the use of synthetic hair dyes. These pages help you make an informed choice about whether to cover up gray, become a blonde, or just go with nature.

THE RISKS

One 1994 American Cancer Society and FDA study found that women who had used black hair dye for more than 20 years had a slightly higher than average risk of death from non-Hodgkins lymphoma and multiple myeloma, a rare, leukemialike disease. Dr. Samuel Epstein and David Steinman, authors of *The Safe Shopper's Bible* (see *Directory,* pages 122-124), also point out a link between lifetime use of permanent and semipermanent hair dyes with an increased risk of non-Hodgkins lymphoma and leukemia.

In another study, carried out in 1993 by the Harvard School of Public Health and the University of Athens Medical School, researchers assessed that the risk of developing ovarian cancer soared 70 percent in women who dye their hair with permanent color 1-4 times a year. Of course, these women may have had other common factors in their lives that caused the cancer. The trouble is, nobody's sure yet. Even temporary dyes and rinses contain colors such as Acid Orange 87, Solvent Brown 44, Avid Blue 178, and Acid Violet 73, which have shown carcinogenic activity. DEA and TEA (see page 16) are also used.

Bleaches are safer than dyes, with fewer, if any long-term risks. The downside of bleach, however, is that it can dry and damage the hair itself, so you need to condition lavishly.

THE NATURAL CHOICE

The good news is that there is an increasing choice of plant-derived colorants that give excellent results, based on natural elements such as henna, marigold, indigo, blue malva, hibiscus, logwood, and chamomile, and which are ever more widely

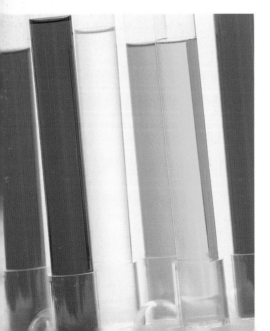

available. Look for dyes by Logona, Rainbow Research Henna, Naturcolor, Urtekram , Herbatint, Igora Botanics, and the Body Shop's Herbal Hair Colorants, which you mix yourself.

If you don't want to color your own hair, discuss your concerns with your hair colorist and ask if they would mind if you brought your own natural dye into the salon for them to use. They will probably be reluctant to guarantee results, but you may nevertheless feel safer leaving the actual technique to the experts. Hairdressers may also be able to offer you a vegetable dye, now widely available in salons – but if you're concerned about avoiding man-made chemicals, ask to see the label: some vegetable dyes contain both vegetable dye *and* chemicals, and so are not as pure as they appear.

The Aveda Shades of Enlightenment Blonding Process mixes a minimum of ammonia and hydrogen-peroxide bleaches with organically grown sunflower, castor, and jojoba oils, but also features a small amount of mineral oil. Daniel Field, meanwhile, is a London-based hairdresser who is pioneering the use of more natural hair colorants in his salon (see *Directory,* pages 122-124), even formulating an alternative to traditional bleaches that include seaweed extracts.

Making your own hair dyes is a sophisticated art, but simple infusions can brighten and deliver depth of color to hair. To enrich your natural shade, try the recipes on pages 86-87.

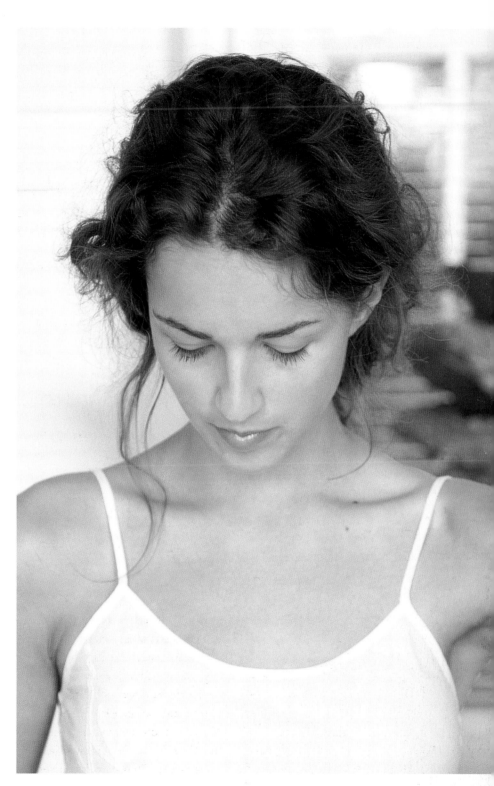

hair color
recipes

Although the results from these home hair-coloring treatments will never be as dramatic as chemical colorants – and will not cover gray – they will make a noticeable difference.

Sage and black tea rinse (for gray hair)

4 tbs dried sage leaves

½ cup (100 ml) water

1 tea bag

Boil the water and make some tea as for drinking, using the sage and the tea bag. Let it stand for 30 minutes. Apply to the hair, leave on for 30 minutes, then rinse. Shampoo and condition the hair as normal.

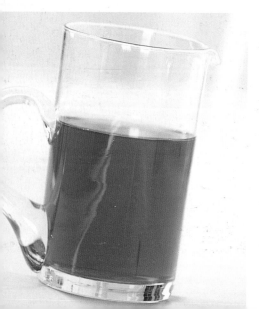

Permanent red rinse

Warning: Henna is a permanent red dye, so be absolutely sure you want to change your color before you try this. Always try a strand test first to establish that the color is as you'd like it to be. Use surgical gloves (from a pharmacy) while carrying out the treatment, since henna stains the skin as well as sinks and bowls. To avoid staining, put an oil-based barrier cream all the way around your hairline before using henna.

1 tea bag or 1 tsp ground coffee

½ cup (100 g) henna powder

1 tbs olive oil

1 cup (200 ml) water

Make a cup of tea or coffee with the water, let it steep, then strain. Add it to a bowl in which you've placed the henna powder. Mix in the olive oil and add more water (if necessary) to make a smooth paste. Immediately apply the preparation to the hair, then cover the hair with plastic wrap. If preferred, you can put another plastic bag over the top and wrap a warm towel around it. Leave on for 2-3 hours, then rinse, shampoo, and condition the hair.

• Cranberry juice can be used as a natural brightener for red hair; it boosts the shine and enhances the red color to make it more vibrant. To use, saturate the hair with cranberry juice before shampooing. Leave the juice on for 2 minutes, then cleanse the hair with a gentle shampoo. Condition the hair as usual.

Rinse for dark hair

4 tbs dried sage

2 tbs dried rosemary

2 cups (400 ml) water

1 tbs cider vinegar

Simmer all the ingredients in a glass saucepan for 30 minutes. Strain and cool, and use as a final rinse for hair.

Alternative rinses for dark hair

• An elderberry rinse will add a subtle mahogany color to dark hair. Put a large handful of elderberries in a pan and cover completely with water. Simmer for 20 minutes, strain, and let it cool. Use as a final rinse after shampooing.

• Adding apple cider vinegar to the final rinse for dark hair improves shine, giving the illusion of more depth to your natural color.

Blonde-boosting rinse

1 cup (200 g) calendula flowers
1 cup (200 g) chamomile flowers
1 cup (200 g) orange peel
½ cup (100 g) lemon peel (if the hair is also oily)
½ cup dried comfrey root
3 cups (600 ml) apple cider vinegar

Use either dried or fresh flowers, and mix all the ingredients together. If you're using fresh herbs, use twice the quantity in each instance. Place them in a very large jar; heat the vinegar to just below boiling point and pour it on the herbs. Put the rinse in a cool, dark place for 10 days, and shake the jar every day. At the end of 10 days, strain the mixture through a piece of cheesecloth, pressing firmly to squeeze out the last of the vinegar. Mix 2 tablespoons of the herb-infused vinegar with 2 cups (400 ml) of warm water and use as a final rinse after shampooing and conditioning.

Easy blonde-brightening rinse

10 chamomile tea bags
4 cups (800 ml) boiling water

Pour the water over the chamomile tea bags and steep them for a few minutes before removing the tea bags. Let the infusion cool before use. After shampooing, pour the brightening infusion over the hair. Use a bowl to catch the rinse and then pour it over the hair two or three more times.

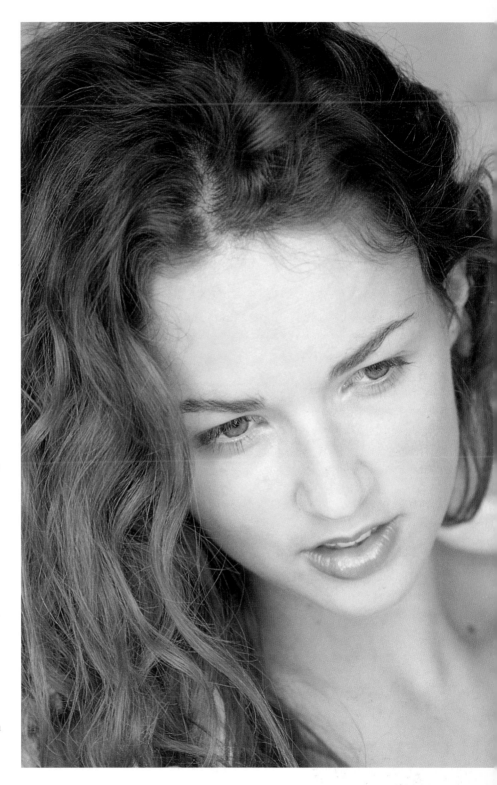

reviving
head massage

Scalp massage has more than one benefit: it stimulates the hair follicles to encourage healthy hair growth and helps combat stress. Follow the steps below to reduce tension in the scalp.

Why is head massage – which is so popular in India and the Orient – so good for hair and our wellbeing? Health practitioners and trichologists can tell a lot about stress levels from the scalp. When we're stressed, the muscles holding the scalp to the skull tighten; in fact, the scalp may hardly move at all if you try to manipulate it. Massage loosens those muscles, which in turn has a relaxing effect, at the same time boosting blood flow.

In Ayurvedic medicine, it is thought that head massage (which is an integral part of this approach to health) energizes the cerebrospinal fluid, strengthening the nervous system.

When oil is applied to the head, it is absorbed by the hair roots; these in turn are connected with the nerve fibers that lead directly to the brain. The oil also strengthens the hair, leaving it glossy as well as easing many scalp disorders, and even reducing,

some believe, baldness. To make sure of the optimal functioning of an infant's brain, mothers in India even keep a piece of cotton or linen soaked in oil on the baby's fontanelle (the soft spot on the top of the head, which is covered at birth only by a membrane) until the bones of the skull close up in the weeks after birth.

HOLISTIC HAIR RESCUE

"Applied directly to the scalp via massage," says botanical beauty expert Philip B., "certain botanical blends can eliminate two of the most common causes of hair loss: dirt- and oil-plugged pores, and poor circulation."

Massaging essential oils into the scalp helps deliver their active benefits directly to the hair follicles and to the scalp itself. It's best to do the massage before bedtime, sleep with your hair wrapped in a towel, then wash and shampoo it the next morning.

Performing a relaxing head massage

You can do this to yourself sitting up, or, better still, ask someone else to do it to you – then return the favor.

1 Stroke lightly from the forehead, over the top of the head and down to the neck. Next start at the temples and stroke over the ears. Repeat the sequence, using firmer strokes.

2 Using the pads of the fingertips, make small but firm circles all over the scalp. Start at the forehead and work back over the whole head. Pay special attention to the areas around the ears and at the base of the skull, where tension often builds up.

3 Don't just move the fingers – move the scalp around as much as possible, to help relax the underlying muscles.

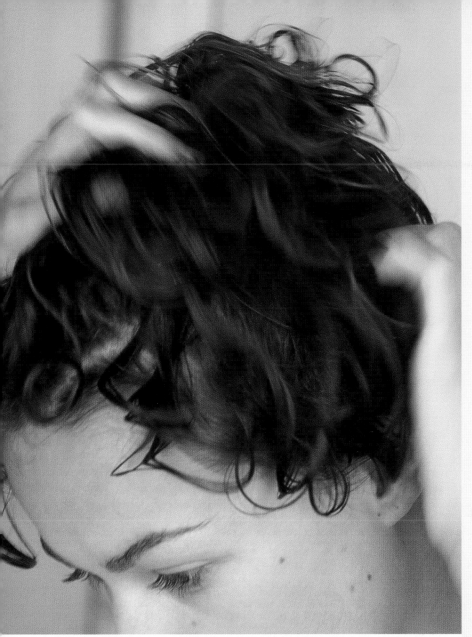

Hair-booster scalp massage oil

Use a base of 2 tbs extra-virgin olive oil, with 1 tbs wheatgerm oil and 1 tbs jojoba oil.

• For dry hair, add 8 drops geranium oil, 12 drops lavender oil, and 6 drops sage oil.

• For oily hair (yes, this really works!), add 8 drops of tea tree oil, 8 drops lavender oil, and 8 drops patchouli oil.

• For normal hair, add 8 drops rose oil, 8 drops lavender oil, and 8 drops rosemary oil.

• For dandruff, add 10 drops of cypress oil, 10 drops of juniper oil, and 8 drops of cedarwood oil.

For best results, heat the oil. You can do this by placing a cup or small pitcher in a bowl of just-boiled hot water. Leave for 5 minutes, and the oil will warm up. (Wrapping hair in a hot towel after the massage also helps the oils penetrate the hair shaft.)

Work the oil through the hair, then carry out a soothing head massage (see left) to calm the entire nervous system. For extra benefits, add in these massage movements:

• Massaging the forehead generates a feeling of wellbeing in the brain and is said to improve eyesight and concentration.

• Massaging the temples improves eyesight and concentration, and creates a "centered" state.

• Massaging the eyebrows and orbital bone relaxes the whole body and is especially beneficial for the eyes and for those who suffer from headaches.

4 Stroke the hair, then lightly clasp a handful of hair from the root area and gently pull the hair upward, away from the scalp.

5 Release the hair, then glide your fingers through it. Build up a rhythm, pulling with one hand, gliding with the other. Imagine the tension flowing out through the ends of your hair.

6 Position your hands on each side of your head, with fingers over the ears and the heels of your hands by the temples.

7 Gently press your hands in and hold for a couple of seconds.

8 Slowly release pressure, glide hands up the sides of the head, and gently off the top. Repeat several times.

eating

for healthy hair

Eat well, and your hair will repay you by gleaming with health. The following hints will help you choose the best foods for healthy hair and show you how to keep it in top condition.

Your hair is what you eat, and if you want lustrous, shiny hair, eating a balanced, organic diet will help feed it with nutrients. Skimping on nutrition, meanwhile, can have a negative impact on your hair's condition.

One of the world's leading hair experts, Philip Kingsley, reports a huge surge in the number of 25- to 35-year-olds coming into his clinic with thinning hair, and poor nutrition is the culprit. He blames leaving long gaps between meals and a calorie intake of under 2,000 per day; excessive exercise can also impact on hair health. According to Kingsley, four-hour-plus lapses between meals on a regular basis can create a drop in energy levels in the hair follicles. He advises carrying fruit as a snack and making sure all meals are well balanced.

Good hair foods include wholegrain bread, nonfat milk, chicken, orange juice, leafy dark vegetables (including kale, spinach, and mustard greens),

and broccoli. Boost your intake of vitamin B2 and biotin by eating more avocados, yeast extract, tomatoes, and egg yolk. Zinc deficiency can also cause dry, flaky scalp (for zinc-rich foods, see page 67.)

In addition, it's important to eat enough of the right fats and oils (see page 67). According to some experts, women on very low-fat diets – in which less than 15 percent of their total daily calorie intake comes from fat – can develop thin, dull hair. If you start to eat well with hair health in mind, however, don't expect overnight miracles. According to Philip Kingsley, "it takes at least three to four months for hair follicles to benefit from nutritional changes, and about six to twelve months before you'll notice a difference in thinning hair."

• For healthy hair, drink at least two cups a day of herbal hair tea that contains such ingredients as rosemary, nettle, and horsetail. Combining them

with other herbs such as peppermint gives a refreshing, pleasant taste.

BEAUTY AND THE BRUSH
Your granny was right: brushing 50-100 strokes stimulates the scalp and helps spread the natural protective oils through the hair. Brushing hair can be a wonderful massage for the scalp, too.

Hairbrushes can be made from many materials, including plastic and synthetics. Seek out those made from natural materials; rubber is much more gentle on the scalp than metal or plastic prongs. The most hair-friendly brushes have prongs that are mounted on a rubber pad, which allows the brush to breathe. If you can find brushes with wooden handles, they are lovely to touch, have a long life, and are also gentle on the scalp. Larger natural food stores often carry a range of wooden brushes. Aveda's are excellent (they're my brushes of choice), and widely available in stores.

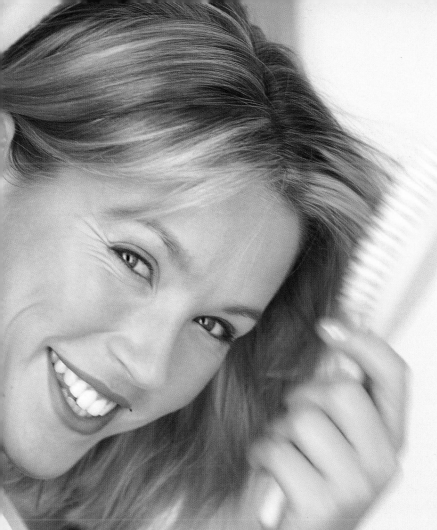

whether someone has taken drugs, it does not seem quite so easy to dismiss the idea that our hair gives clues to what we have and haven't eaten, drunk, or otherwise consumed.

WELL-NOURISHED HAIR

Of course, the best way to make sure your hair is being adequately nourished is to eat a varied, fresh organic diet, rich in wholegrains, fruit, and vegetables, and with minimum of sugar and alcohol. Before you submit to hair analysis – usually an expensive vitamin and mineral supplement regime will be recommended to combat your hair imbalances – eat as healthily as you can over a period of several months, and then see how your hair gleams, your skin glows with good health, and your energy level surges.

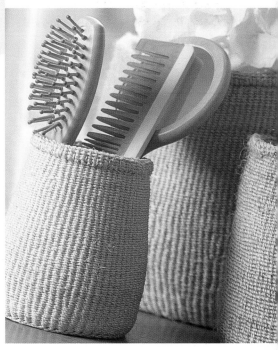

HAIR ANALYSIS – AND WHAT IT TELLS YOU

Can your hair tell an expert whether you have a nutritional deficiency? Many complementary therapists believe so, although doctors are still skeptical. If you have hair problems – thinning or lackluster hair – this may be linked with a nutritional deficiency: for example, brittle hair can indicate a copper or calcium imbalance. Because what we eat, drink, and otherwise ingest is laid down in our hair, it is thought by some to be an indicator of what our diet is lacking. Think of a

quarry, and how the different ages are represented by different strata of minerals. Hair is rather like that.

Many physicians still regard hair analysis as "nutritional quackery" (to quote one website), saying that there are no vitamins in the hair, except in the root below the scalp, and that it's not possible to identify mineral deficiencies because lower limits of "normal" minerals in the hair have not been scientifically established. However, when taking into consideration that hair analysis is increasingly used by law courts to tell

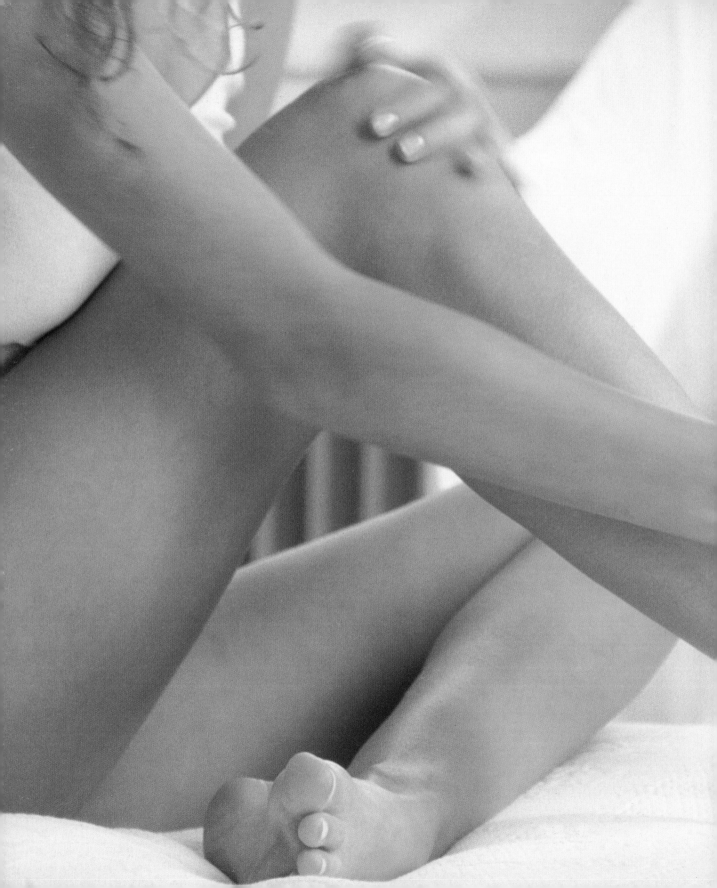

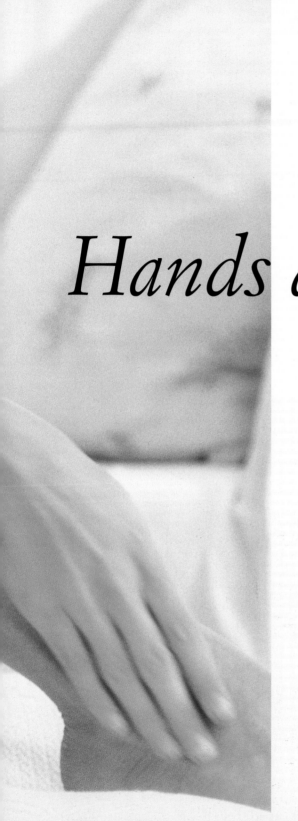

Hands and feet

Hands and feet are often low down the beauty priority list, the forgotten extremities. Yet, just like hair, the health, condition, and grooming of your feet and hands tell the world a lot about how you feel about yourself as well as your general wellbeing. Happy, cared-for feet also make for a happy person, especially when you consider they may carry us up to 70,000 miles in a lifetime. Consider the organic options that put healthy and pretty fingers and toes within everyone's reach.

destress
hand exercises

Hands are one of our most important features, used in every aspect of our life. To give yourself strong, supple hands, follow these tips regularly – you will feel the difference.

More important than hands that look glamorous or feel like velvet is to have flexible, strong hands whose joints will not stiffen and seize up in old age.

RELEASING TENSION

Hands, and particularly fingers, are a prime area of the body for holding tension. If you destress your hands you can, in effect, destress your whole being and restore a sense of calm and balance. Make a conscious effort during the day of checking to see whether you've unwittingly clenched your hands into tight fists. If you catch yourself clenching your fists, shake your hands vigorously for 30 seconds to release tension.

Meanwhile to keep hands in good shape, do the following exercises which will maintain strength and supplenenss all life long. First, warm your hands up with a massage oil (see page 102).

Exercising your hands

1 Clench the fists tightly and hold for three seconds; then fling the fingers open, spacing and stretching them for a further three counts.

2 Repeat the sequence 10 times, then rotate the wrists both ways 10 times.

3 Curl the fingers one after another to make a loose fist, palms down. Slowly turn palms upward and gently unfurl the fingers one by one , stretching and relaxing them as you go. Repeat the exercise five times on each hand to achieve the maximum benefit from the exercise.

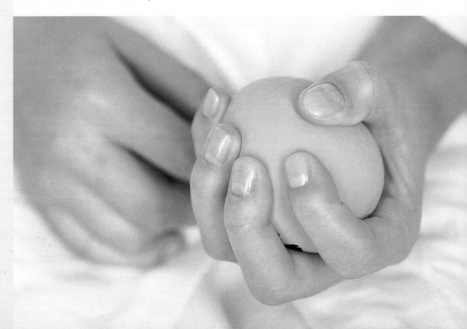

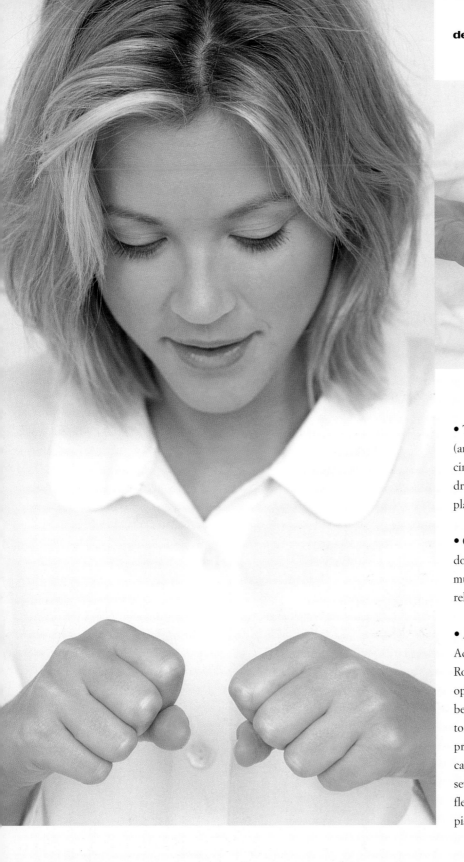

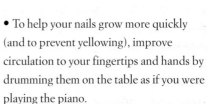

• To help your nails grow more quickly (and to prevent yellowing), improve circulation to your fingertips and hands by drumming them on the table as if you were playing the piano.

• Origins makes a "stress ball" that offers double benefits: it not only exercises the muscles of the hands, it is also effective at relieving stress.

• Alternatively, try piano lessons. According to a spokesman at Britain's Royal Academy of Music, although the optimum age to begin piano lessons is between seven and ten, "it is never too late to take up piano – which definitely promotes suppleness and strength. People can successfully play piano through their seventies and eighties, with great flexibility." You may never be a concert pianist – but your hands will love you for it.

handcare
recipes

Hands and nails always suffer most from harsh weather and heavy work, such as gardening and cleaning. So here's how to pamper and polish your hands – as naturally as possible.

There are some wonderful all-natural hand creams on the market. Weleda, Jurlique, Logona, Dr. Hauschka, and Living Nature (see *Directory,* pages 122-124) make excellent, entirely pure creams, but here are some inexpensive alternatives that put back what everyday life takes out of your hands.

• If nails are discolored, clean them with lemon juice and scrub them in white wine vinegar.

• Mix a teaspoonful of honey with two teaspoonfuls of almond or olive oil, and massage into hands after washing and drying. Put on a pair of cotton gloves and sleep in

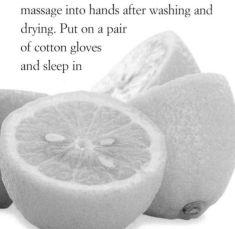

the treatment. Wash your hands in the morning (best on those nights when you're sleeping alone!)

• The perfect nail is strong but flexible so it doesn't snap when life throws challenges at your hands. Most nail hardeners work by drying out the nail's vital oils, making them brittle. Soaking your nails daily in warm almond or olive oil (which can be used over and over) is the ultimate strengthener. Then wipe the hands clean – or better still, massage the oil left on the skin until it sinks in. (You can store the leftover oil for reuse time and again.)

• Each time you apply a hand treatment, give yourself a mini-hand massage to help the moisturizers penetrate and to encourage good circulation in your extremities. Cradle one hand in the other and firmly massage the palm with the other thumb, using deep, circular movements. Turn the hand over and gently work around the joints and in

between the fingers to loosen any stiffness. Carefully pull and relax each finger, then use slight pressure to ease it backward away from the palm. Finish by using the thumb and fingers of the other hand to stroke down each finger firmly from the tips as far as the wrist, to decongest the entire hand.

• If you wear nail polish, there's no alternative: you must use polish remover. Most are very drying, but adding a few drops of almond oil to the bottle of polish remover helps put back some of the oil that the polish-stripper takes out (shake well before each use.) Always choose polish-remover that is acetone-free, which avoids the worst of the offenders.

• As an alternative to wearing commercial nail polish, try buffing your nails with beeswax or cocoa butter and a soft cloth.

• Organic gardening may be good for our health and for the planet's health, but it's the enemy of smooth, soft hands. Gloves, however, make it hard to feel roots in the ground and make performing tasks clumsy. The best solution I've found is to wear surgeons' latex gloves, available from pharmacies; you can feel everything in the soil, but they keep hands dry and perfectly clean. Be warned, though: they won't withstand sharp thorns or stinging plants.

• Minimize the exposure of hands to all kinds of chemicals. Water, soap, and household cleaners dry out your hands, also predisposing them to painful hangnails: small pieces of detached skin at the side or base of your nail that tend to snag on clothing and towels, and rank alongside paper cuts as minor but incredibly annoying skin problems. Make sure to wear protective gloves (try the latex gloves mentioned above) when doing household chores such as washing dishes, floors, windows, or cleaning the bathtub, in fact any work that involves the use of chemical cleaning fluids.

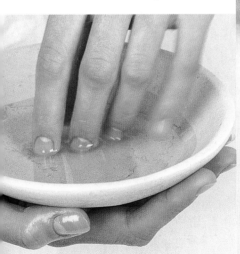

Rich lemon hand cream

juice of one freshly squeezed lemon

almond oil

1 tsp beeswax

5 drops lemon oil

Strain the lemon juice through cheesecloth. Pour the juice into a measuring cup and add an equal amount of almond oil. Melt the beeswax in a ovenproof bowl over a pan of hot water. The almond oil will be floating on top of the lemon juice; scoop off some of the oil and add to the beeswax, stirring, until the wax has melted. Add the rest of the contents of the measuring cup; heat, shake, and stir until blended. Stir until cool with the wooden spoon and add the lemon oil, drop by drop. Transfer to a jar, and shake occasionally until the cream is cold.

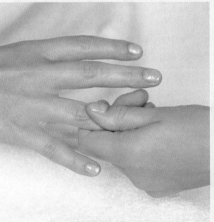

Cuticle softener

1 organic egg yolk

1 tbs pineapple juice

5 drops lemon juice

1 drop lemon essential oil

Mix the egg with the pineapple juice and add the lemon juice and lemon oil.

Soak nails in this mixture for 15 minutes, and push the cuticles back gently with an orangewood stick.

Tough-as-nails aromatherapy oil

⅛ cup (25 ml) jojoba oil

½ tsp sweet almond oil

5 drops lavender essential oil

5 drops frankincense essential oil

This makes a moisturizing, lightly antiseptic oil that can be massaged into nails morning and night to keep them flexible but strong, and it moisturizes cuticles, too.

Winter hand saver

When the central heating goes on and winter winds start to blow, hands become drier than usual. The natural graininess of sugar in this mixture exfoliates beautifully, while olive oil is one of nature's great skin softeners.

1 tbs organic granulated sugar

2 tbs olive oil

3 drops of your favorite essential oils

Combine the ingredients in a small bowl, and dip your fingers into the oil, massaging it gently into rough, red skin, calluses, cuticles, and knuckles, all the way up beyond the wrist joint. Sit and let the mixture sink in for as long as you like, before removing with a towel that has been soaked in hot water. Dry your hands and drench them in moisturizer.

Try performing this treatment in the bathtub, where you can sit still for as long as you like. Just remember to keep your hands above the water level.

nail foods *and natural polish*

Having elegantly painted nails can give you instant confidence, but truly natural nail polish does not exist. So if you want a high-gloss, colorful manicure, be informed about your choices.

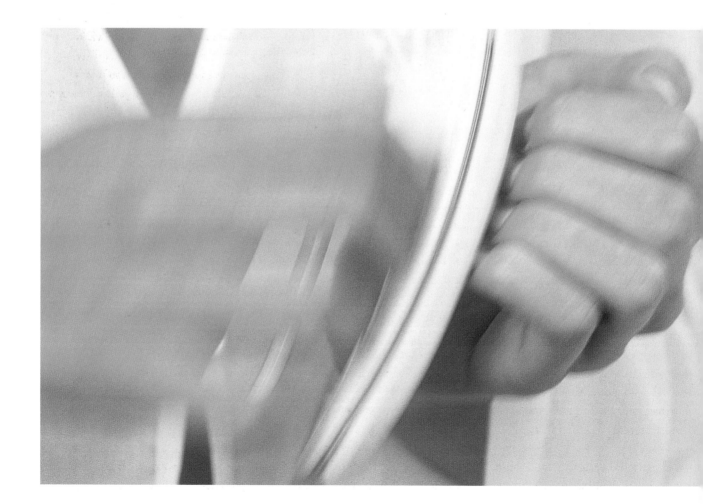

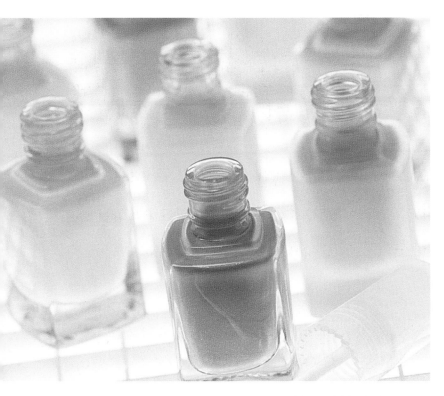

Increasingly, nail-polish manufacturers are leaving certain chemicals out of their formulations. According to the American International Agency for Research on Cancer, toluene and formaldehyde, both widely used as preservatives and bonding agents in cosmetic polishes, can cause nose and throat irritation, rashes, headaches, nausea, and asthma. What's more, according to experts, formaldehyde is a known carcinogen. Even though painting your nails hardly qualifies as the "extreme exposure" that brings real risk, natural health advice is to minimize contact with these chemicals.

Manufacturers, including Avon and Clinique, are now formulating their polishes without these chemicals, often proclaiming the polishes to be "toluene- and formaldehyde-free" on the labels (otherwise, scan the ingredient list.) Even so, it only takes a whiff to tell you that even "natural" polishes contain strong chemicals, so you may prefer to buff your nails to a shine rather than rely on polish. And if you do use polish, avoid applying makeup or touching your skin until the polish has dried, or you may risk skin irritation. In the meantime, watch out for news of a revolutionary "green" polish, the result of research by French scientists, based entirely on water and safe enough for use even by children, who are attracted at an ever younger age to painted fingers and toes.

Look for nail polish removers that are "acetone-free"; acetone is extremely drying to nails. The London natural pharmacy, Farmacia, has produced a natural nail-care line that includes gentler polish removers (see *Directory,* pages 122-124).

Think hard before you use a nail hardener, meanwhile. Nail hardeners, which feature harsh chemicals, work by drying out the nail, making it tough – yet prone to breaking. The best treatment you can give your nails is each night, before bedtime, to anoint your cuticles with oil (see page 96). The massage action boosts circulation, while the oils condition the nail, resulting in improved flexibility – so your fingernails don't snap when challenged by such tasks as filing, gardening, and carrying suitcases.

Be sure to store nail polish removers well out of the reach of children. Many contain acetronile, which breaks down into cyanide when swallowed. Likewise, all nail polishes should be kept out of children's way.

EATING FOR HEALTHIER NAILS
Nails need the same nutrients as skin and hair – and if your diet falls short, your nails will show it. A common cause of brittle nails is thought to be iron deficiency. Too little vitamin A and calcium also cause nail dryness and brittleness, while an inadequate intake of B vitamins results in excessive dryness and nail fragility.

Tiny white spots that move up the nail as it grows out can signal zinc deficiency. For details of foods you can eat to help combat these nail problems, see pages 66-67.

natural
manicure

Take some time for yourself and perform this gentle step-by-step manicure. The information given here shows you how to achieve good results, while limiting environmental impact.

How to do a manicure

1 If you are going to use nail polish or remover, open the windows before starting to minimize your exposure to the chemicals. In addition, ask at your usual beauty-supply store or pharmacy for acetone-free polish remover; alternatively, look for the words "gentle" or "non-drying" on the label, which are clues.

2 Remove old nail polish: use a cotton pad and (for the tiny bits) a cuticle stick that has been wrapped in absorbent cotton. Never use a wooden or metal instrument on your nails unless it has been carefully buffered with cotton first.

3 Shorten any nails that need cutting down – using nail scissors in preference to clippers, which can cause cracks. Cut from the side to the

middle of the nail. Then shape the nails with an emery board, stroking lightly from the edges of the nail toward the center. The softer and springier the emery board, the better. Look for the kinds that are almost squishy to touch, thanks to their foam backing, and last virtually a lifetime.

4 Using a dropper, apply Tough-As-Nails Aromatherapy Oil (see recipe page 97) to the cuticle area, and massage in thoroughly with circular movements of the thumb.

5 Soak the fingertips in a bowl of warm water for at least a minute and dry thoroughly afterward.

6 Gently push back the skin around the cuticles, working at the dead skin to create a neat, clean line. Use a cuticle stick wrapped in cotton or, better still, a rubber-tipped "hoof stick."

7 Wash the hands thoroughly and brush the nails with a soft nail brush. Rinse the nails and dry them carefully on a towel. If you are going to apply polish, be aware that even a tiny amount of moisture or oil will spoil your manicure by preventing the polish from sticking to the nail. If you are simply going to buff your nails, apply another dot of oil and work into the nail surface, then buff with a nail buffer. You can use one made of chamois; alternatively, The Body Shop makes an excellent, springy buffer. To buff the nail, always work in an up-and-down motion, rather than side to side across the nail. This stimulates blood flow and delivers a beautiful sheen.

8 If using polish, brush on a protective base coat to cover the entire nail surface, stopping short of the cuticle. A base coat keeps colored polish from staining nails.

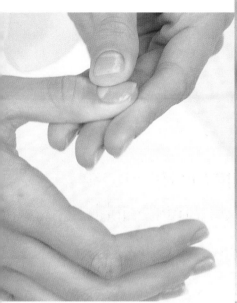

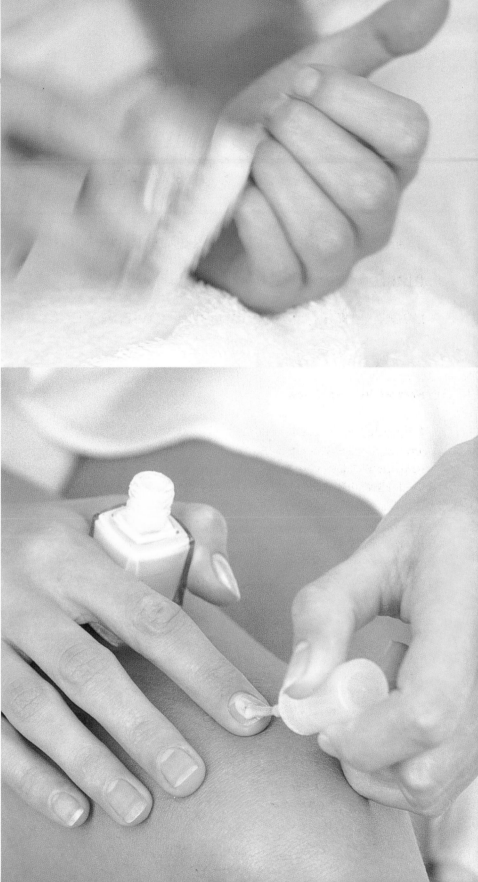

9 Apply two coats of your chosen toluene- and formaldehyde-free nail color, starting with a stroke down the center of the nail and then a stroke on each side, being careful to avoid the cuticle. (If you do smudge the polish, dip an orangewood stick in remover and carefully wipe away.)

10 Lightly brush on one layer of top coat to add gloss and protect against chipping and abrasion. When nails are dry to the touch, add a drop of your Tough-As-Nails oil (see recipe page 97) to each cuticle and rub it very lightly onto the surface of the polish; it acts as an amazingly effective quick dry. Ideally, however, you should allow half an hour for your nails to be completely dry, so allow yourself at least 30 minutes of pure relaxation.

11 To prolong the life of your manicure, brush on a fresh topcoat every other day.

relaxing
foot massage

Treating weary feet to a massage is the next best thing to an all-over body massage; as you knead each foot, with its thousands of nerve endings, the day's angst just melts away.

What you need

Soft, warm hands Make sure your hands are not cold or rough to the touch. Prepare your hands by rubbing in massage oil to soften and warm your fingers and palms.

Light massage oil So that your hands can move over your feet without sticking, a light massage oil is essential. To make a light oil, try mixing a couple of tablespoons of almond oil with two to three drops of jasmine or lavender essential oil.

A warm environment Make sure the room is warm and comfortable; being barefoot in a cold room will prevent you from relaxing completely.

A bath towel Place a towel across your knees and one under your feet to absorb any stray oil.

The technique

1 Stroke down the left foot from the toes to the ankle, using both hands. Then glide your hands back up to the toes. Repeat until the foot feels warm and relaxed.

2 Supporting the left ankle on your right knee, use your right hand to hold the ball of the foot and gently rotate the foot twice one way and then twice the other.

3 Continue to rest your left ankle on your right knee. Grasp the toes with your right hand and move them gently back and forth a few times to loosen them up.

4 Run your thumbs up the four "grooves" on top of the foot, which start between each toe. Stroke each "groove" firmly with both thumbs at least twice.

5 Using the middle and index fingers, make small, firm rotations all over the ankle area.

6 Supporting the left foot with your left hand, use your right thumb and index finger to work on the toes. Starting with the little toe, stroke, make circular movements, and gently pull each toe. Repeat the sequence three times. Now clasp all the toes together and pull gently.

7 Applying pressure to the sole is very therapeutic. To feel the benefit, continue to rest your left ankle on the right knee. Cradle the left foot with your right hand, fingers on top, thumb on the sole. Starting at the base of the middle toe, apply firm pressure, at half-inch intervals from the center of the sole to the base of the heel. Glide your thumb back to the starting position, then repeat this movement three times.

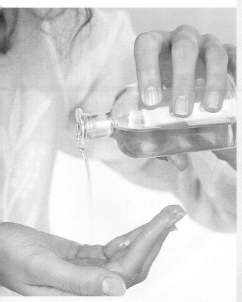

8 To maximize relaxation, rest your left ankle on your right knee and support it still further by holding it with your left hand. Place the fleshy pad of your right hand on the sole of your foot, in the arch, with your fingers on top of the foot. Press firmly, maintaining the pressure for a few seconds, then releasing. Repeat four times for maximum benefit.

9 To finish, repeat movement **1**. Then change legs and reverse the positions.

Note: If someone else is performing the massage for you, adapt the movements slightly, so they can be performed with your foot resting comfortably on a pillow in their lap.

Two-minute foot treat For instant refreshment during the day, take off your shoes, rub your feet, and circle the ankles.

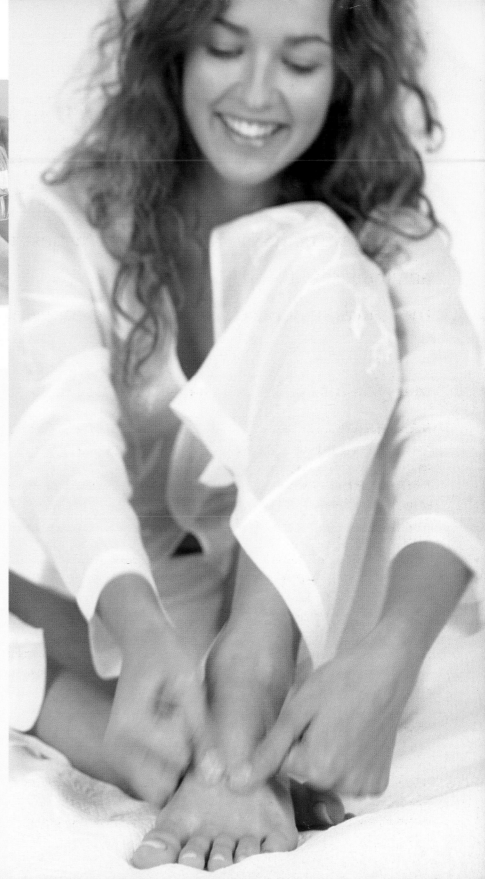

footcare
recipes

Feet can be sandal-worthy all year with just a little effort on a weekly basis. Take the strain off the body's most neglected area by indulging in the foot and leg treats described below.

10 steps to gorgeous feet

1 Cut nails straight across – shaping can result in ingrown nails.

2 Apply Tough-As-Nails Cuticle Oil (see page 97), or Dr. Hauschka's Neem Oil.

3 Soak your feet in a plastic bowl of lukewarm water, with a few drops of invigorating essential oil well blended into the water. Peppermint cools, chamomile softens, and lavender heals.

4 Apply cuticle softener (for an effective homemade version see page 97); wait a minute or two, and then gently push back cuticles with a rubber "hoof" stick or an orangewood stick wrapped in absorbent cotton. Do not cut the cuticle skin; leave that to salon professionals. Do not be tempted to push back the cuticles so far that they reveal the little moon: the cuticle protects the nail bed, which is a mass of

blood vessels and is very swift to show signs of damage.

5 Slough off dead skin with a pumice stone or a foot scrubber.

6 Massage the feet with a rich cream or oil to stimulate, relax, and help flexibility. (See pages 102-103 for more details on foot massage.)

7 If you are going to use polish, clean the nails with soapy water and dry thoroughly.

8 If you don't have any toe-separators, which salons use for pedicures, cheat by separating your toes by placing rolled-up tissues between your toes, or cotton balls. Otherwise, it is easy to smudge the polish.

9 Apply a base coat, polish, and then top coat. Work from the little toe to the big

toe, applying from the bottom of nails to the tips. Apply two coats of color, waiting a minute in between to allow the first layer to dry. In winter, you may prefer to let your nails breathe by skipping nail polish altogether.

10 If you are in a hurry, apply a tiny drop of Tough-As-Nails Cuticle Oil (see page 97), or any type of vegetable oil, which will harden the polish fast. If not, enjoy the opportunity to put your feet up while your nails dry!

PEBBLE FOOTBATH
When giving yourself a footbath, place marbles or pebbles in the bottom of a plastic bowl, then move your feet back and forth over the stones as you soak. Exercise your feet and toes by picking up the rocks and rolling them forward and then backward.

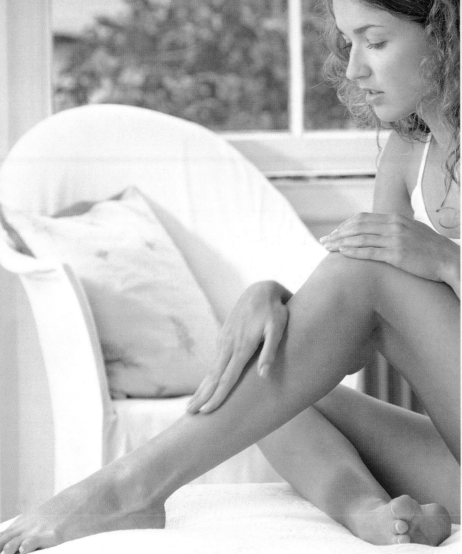

Rosemary-mint-zing foot tonic

1 cup (200 ml) whole organic milk
5 sprigs fresh rosemary, including the
stems
1 cup fresh mint leaves
2 tsp peppermint extract or 10 drops
peppermint essential oil

Gently simmer the milk with the herbs for about 15 minutes. Remove from the heat and let it cool; strain the mixture and then add the peppermint extract or essential oil.

To use the foot tonic, soak two washcloths or dishtowels in the mixture and wrap them around your feet. Put your feet up and relax for 30 minutes. For maximum relaxation and revival, follow with an oil-rich foot massage (see pages 102-103) before you get back on your feet.

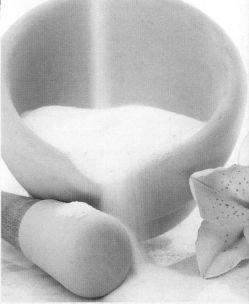

Seaside foot scrub

1 cup sand
1 tbs sea salt
1 tbs powdered dulse seaweed
1 tbs powdered kelp
1 cup (200 ml) olive oil

Mix the dry ingredients together in a preserving jar with an airtight, hinged lid. Then pour in the olive oil and stir well. Apply to the soles of the feet in a circular scrubbing motion, paying particular attention to areas of hard skin. (Add 6 drops of peppermint oil for extra freshness.)

Mask for flaky winter legs

1 avocado
1 banana
1 tbs thick cream
1 tbs sweet almond or avocado oil

Mash all the ingredients together until they form an ultra-smooth paste; then, when you're in the bathtub, apply the paste to cover both the shins and knees, which often become dry and flaky in winter. Keep your legs raised out of the water for about 10 minutes, with the mask on, before rinsing it off.

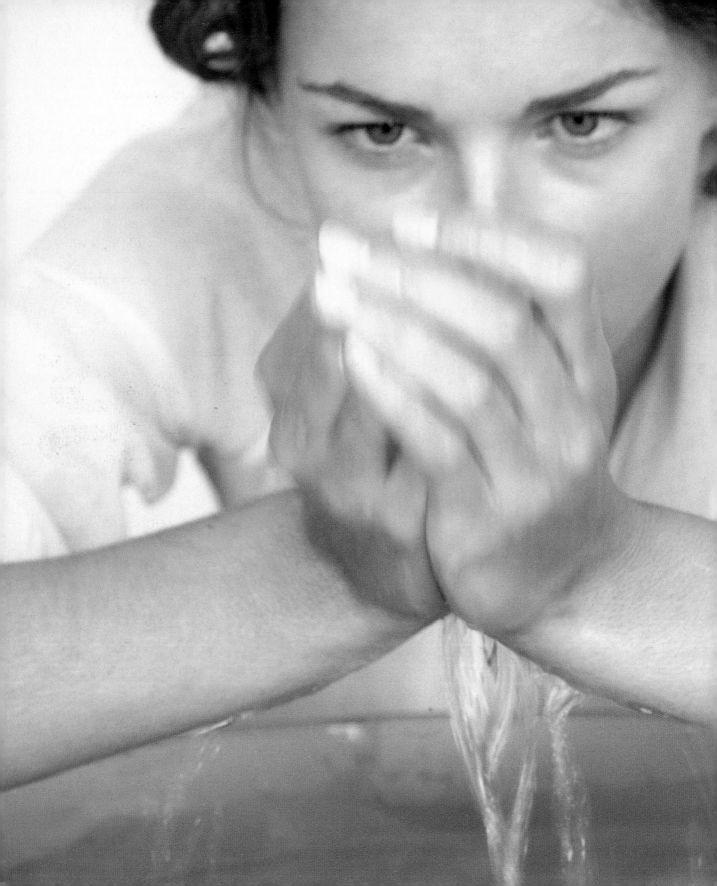

Bathing and bodycare are important daily rituals that put back some of what a stressful life takes out. There is nothing more pleasurable than a relaxing soak at the end of the day. As the skin is

Organic bathing

the body's largest organ and readily absorbs ingredients applied to its surface, you may wish to consider organic bath and bodycare. Today, back-to-nature, botanical bathroom bliss is an option with effective, fragrant, and often mood-lifting and enhancing treats to buy and make.

organic
body treats

A bath is one of the most blissful of all beauty treatments – relax in a tub infused with the scent of herbs or have a long soak in warm water sprinkled with aromatic essential oils.

The first time I started to question the potential impact of cosmetics on my body was after slathering myself in a fabulous, highly perfumed lotion. Five minutes later, it had sunk in. I asked myself: "Where did it go?" Some, I knew (the water and alcohol elements, mostly) had evaporated, but the rest had gone into my skin. Of that, who knows how much had entered my bloodstream, without first being filtered by the liver.

The large surface area of body skin means that you're potentially exposed to a much higher level of chemicals than via, say, your light nightly dab of eye cream. (The sheer speed with which you get through a bottle of body lotion should tell you that.)

Take as a starting point of things to avoid the list on page 16: *10 Ingredients You Don't Want in Your Cosmetics*. As a shortcut, look to the following companies, which make all-natural, synthetic-preservative-free body products: Weleda, Dr. Hauschka, Green People's Company, Living Nature, Burt's Bees, Lavera, and Logona, among others.

Alternatively, instead of creams, try infusing the bath or moisturizing the body with oils such as jojoba, almond, or grapeseed, to which a few drops of essential oils have been added. That way, you will avoid the long list of preservatives that go into many body creams and lotions, since blends based exclusively on oils don't need them to stay uncontaminated. Some essential oils also act as natural preservatives.

Basic recipes for body oils are listed in this chapter. Once you get the hang of mixing them (and it really couldn't be simpler), you can create blends using your favorite aromatherapy oils.

Make sure your bottles are kept away from sunlight to maximize their shelf life and to prevent the oils from becoming rancid.

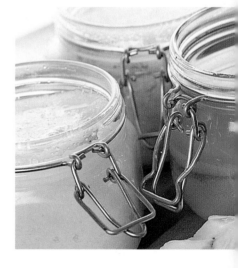

BATHROOM BLISS

For many of us, the bathroom is one place where we can lock the door, stop the world, and escape, yet all too often, a bath becomes just another everyday task on life's "To Do" list. For many, the bath has given way to shortcut showering, instead.

Physiologically, the relaxing effects of soaking in water are easy to understand: warm water displaces weight, making you feel light. As your capillaries dilate from its warmth, your blood pressure drops. What's more, according to Diane Ackerman, author of *A Natural History of the Senses*, a soak in the tub is a "ritual that is restorative, sensuous, religious, or calming."

Anything you use to enhance the ritual can only help nudge you toward aquatic nirvana. A bath can be sheer, indulgent pleasure, but it can also be easily supercharged into something that is more than mere liquid refreshment, by tailoring your ritual to boost energy, relax, recharge, or deliver a sense of stillness in a mad, mad world.

The good news is that the bathtub is one zone where it couldn't be easier to go organic. Instead of foams, which are detergent-based (and usually dry the skin), switch to fragrant oils. Used to infuse baths, they can help with improving your mood while replenishing your skin at the same time. Many aromatherapy companies offer premixed bath blends based on pure vegetable oils and essential oils, and oils, as a rule, don't need to have preservatives added to them. However, be sure to check the label and make sure there's no mineral oil in the recipe.

In natural food stores, entirely natural soaps are now more widely available, made from hardened fats and oils, and fragranced with plant elements; some are even organically based. (Making your own soap is more complicated than many other products for the bath, but in the *Directory,* see pages 122-124, where you'll find the author's recommendation of a soap recipe book.) Look for bath salts – crystal or Dead Sea salt – to which blends of aromatherapy oils have been added.

Alternatively try bath oils, soaks, bath "teas," and salts (see page 111).

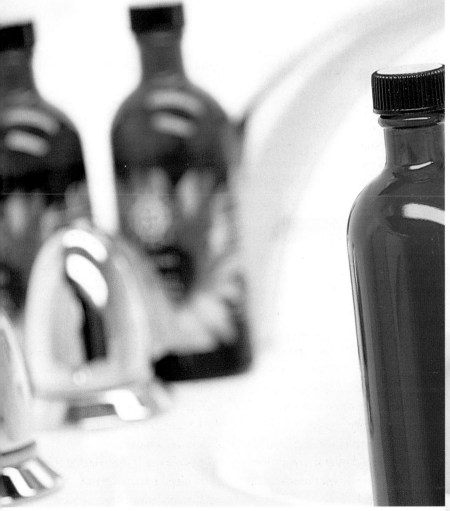

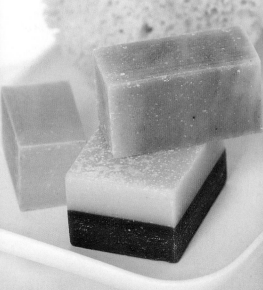

fragrant
bath bags and salts

The bath is the ultimate place to harness the spirit-lifting benefits of herbs and mineral salts. Follow these instructions to make bath bags and salts using your favorite ingredients.

Herbs, tossed directly into water, make for messy bathing, but you can still experience their benefits by making simple bath bags to contain them.

MAKING A BATH BAG

Take an 8 in- (20 cm-) square of cheesecloth, and pile the herbs in the middle. Make a pouch and tie the neck with a long piece of natural string. Tie the string again, in a loop this time. The bag can be hung over the faucet so that the running water is infused with herbs.

If you put a handful of organic oatmeal in the bags, you can use the wet bag to scrub your body, gently exfoliating the skin.

Once you have mastered the art of making bath bags, you can experiment with different recipes, using either fresh or dried organic herbs in numerous combinations. Here are several suggestions to get your imagination started.

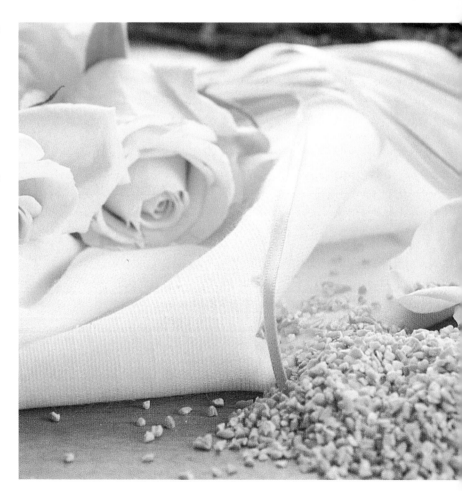

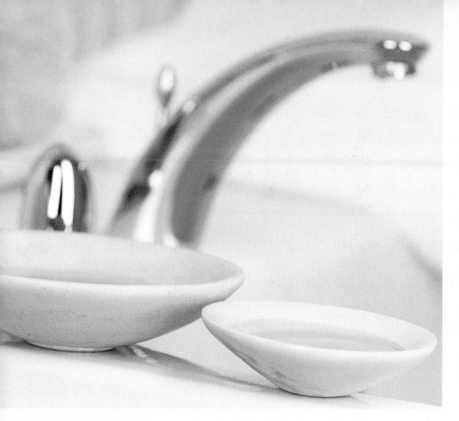

Basic bath salts

Among the big perfume houses, there's a return to once-humble bath salts. They not only neutralize the trace elements that harden water, but also help to remineralize skin; you can make your own, very easily, without any synthetic fragrances. Any combination of essential oils can be used – provided you don't exceed the number of drops used here – but this blend will revive and refresh, giving a boost to tired-looking skin.

12 drops cajuput essential oil

12 drops lavender essential oil

12 drops lemongrass essential oil

8 drops eucalyptus essential oil

1 cup (200 g) coarse or fine salt

1 cup (200 g) Epsom salts

¼ cup (50 ml) glycerin

Combine the oils in a small bowl. In a separate bowl, mix the salts and glycerin until well blended. Stir the essential oil blend into the salt-and-glycerin mixture, and let it stand for 15 minutes. Transfer the salts to a glass container (a dark one, if you don't plan to use the salts up in the next week or so, and they will stay fresh for up to a year.) This recipe makes enough for about four baths.

• By varying the temperature of the bathtub water, you can tailor your bath to be more therapeutic than merely luxurious. For a sedative effect, bathtub water should be 99-102° F (37-39° C) which relaxes and temporarily lowers blood pressure. A bath at 97° F (36° C) is stimulating, because it recharges the central nervous system. (Thermometers can be found in some baby-supply stores, or you can use a kitchen thermometer!)

Invigorating bath bag

1 oz (25 g) rosemary

½ oz (10 g) peppermint

½ cup coarse oatmeal

Summertime bath bag

1 oz (25 g) rose petals

1 oz (25 g) lavender buds

½ cup (75 g) coarse oatmeal

Recovery bath bag

2 tbs dried chamomile flowers

2 tbs dried rosebuds

2 tbs dried lavender flowers

2 tbs dried hop flowers (optional)

Ultra-relaxing bath oil

¼ cup (50 ml) sweet almond oil

10 drops sandalwood oil

5 drops each jasmine oil and orange oil

Decant the almond oil into a bottle and add the essential oils, drop by drop. Shake well until blended, and swish 1 tablespoon of the blend into a bathtub full of warm water.

Variations of bath oil

This basic bath oil recipe can be adapted, depending on your state of mind. To clear the head use the following oils with an almond oil base (as in the Ultra-Relaxing Bath Oil):

10 drops patchouli

5 drops ylang-ylang

5 drops rosemary

When your nerves are on edge after a stressful day, try:

10 drops rose

5 drops lavender

5 drops chamomile

To wake yourself up, try:

10 drops grapefruit oil

5 drops lemon oil

5 drops juniper oil

body
scrubs *and soaks*

The combined power of exercise and body scrubbing are the two most effective ways to boost the circulation and exfoliate the skin, leaving it smooth to the touch and glowing with health.

One of the fastest ways to have gleaming, healthy skin is to buff it with a brush or a natural scrub. Body skin is tougher than that on the face, and while I don't recommend facial exfoliants (except the use of a cheesecloth washcloth, to exfoliate the face on a gentle, daily basis), I find that scrubbing the body with oil-infused salt has it gleaming in no time. What's more, by removing the dead, dry surface skin cells, it's easier for body creams and lotions to do their moisturizing duty.

BEAUTIFUL BRUSHWORK

Body brushing performed twice daily gives maximum results to get your body glowing. Top models swear by its power to slough away dead skin cells and boost circulation; after just a couple of minutes of brushing, you'll literally feel the same sense of exhilaration as after if you'd just taken a brisk 20-minute walk. Some experts

believe it can help banish cellulite, too, by encouraging the elimination of toxins through the lymphatic system and thereby helping to break down fatty pockets.

Use a loofah mitt or a long-handled back brush (the Body Shop's is excellent). With long, upward, sweeping movements, start at the feet and work up the legs and across the hips, bottom, and tummy. Move to the arms: beginning at the hands, move up the arms to the shoulders. With all body brushing, you should always working toward the heart. Avoid the breast area, though, or you risk soreness.

For best results, resist the temptation to pummel your thighs hard, or you can break tiny capillaries. If you have sensitive skin, wet a loofah mitt and use it in the bathtub or shower, instead; the water minimizes any damage by decreasing friction. Get into the habit of brushing twice a day,

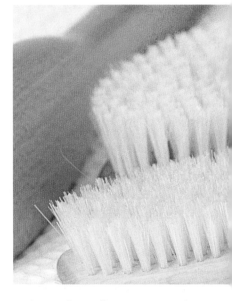

and your skin will soon start to gleam.

Be aware, however, that not all body brushes are created equal. If you have delicate skin, choose a brush with softer bristles – too hard a brush will only bruise the skin and damage capillaries. Whisk the brush against the back of your hand to check that the bristles are firm but not painful.

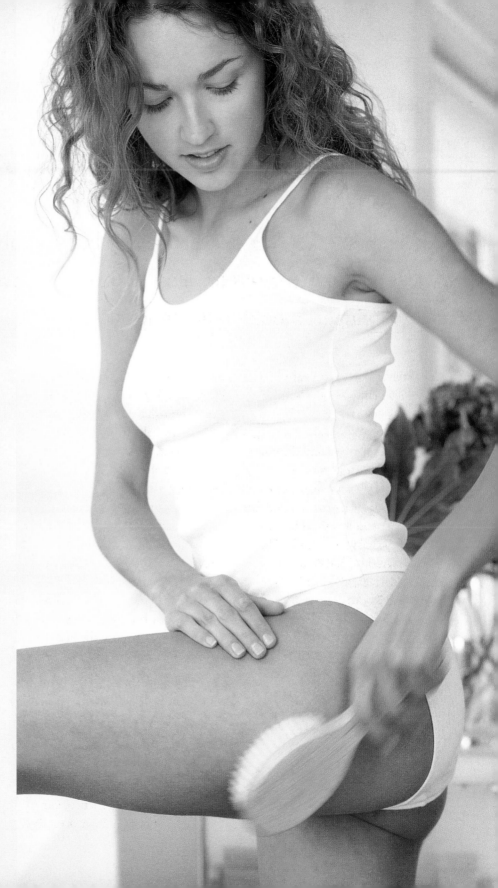

Strawberry-almond-egg body scrub

Strawberries are cleansing and skin-conditioning, while almonds exfoliate and stimulate the skin. Use this mixture for your body only, not your face – nut-based exfoliants can sometimes damage facial skin, which is more fragile. Eggs give a lovely creamy texture to this scrub, making it a real pleasure to use.

½ cup (50 g) chopped cucumber, with skin)

5 hulled strawberries

Just over 2 tbs yogurt – if you have oily skin, use non-fat yogurt, while if your skin is dry, use heavy cream instead

1 tbs baking soda

1 egg

¾ cup (80 g) ground almonds

In a blender, purée the cucumber and the strawberries until really smooth. Add the yogurt, baking soda, egg, and blend on medium-low speed for 20 seconds. Add the almonds and blend on the lowest setting for 2 minutes. Apply to damp skin in a gentle circular motion – always scrubbing gently, to avoid damaging the skin. Rinse thoroughly, then moisturize.

Salt body buff

2 cups (300 g) coarse sea salt

1 cup (200 ml) grapeseed, almond, or olive oil

12-16 drops of essential oil (jasmine or chamomile for a soothing blend)

Pour the salt into an airtight preserving jar with a hinged, sealable lid. Add the essential oils to the cup of base oil, drop by drop, and blend. Then pour into the jar and top up the mix with base oil. Seal the lid and shake well.

body
oils & powders

Making your own body treats can be incredibly satisfying. Create homemade body oils to nourish the skin, and make silky homemade powder to dust on after bathing.

Powder feels good on the skin, helps us get dry fast after a swim or a bath, and is useful in hot weather to stop clothes and shoes from chafing. Most body powders, however, are made of talc, which is related to asbestos and may be potentially carcinogenic. One area where you should be careful about using talc is around the genital area, because of a link with an increased risk of ovarian cancer. As one gynecologist explained to me, "The vagina is designed to act like a vacuum, and talc can easily be absorbed into the body if placed in this area." Switch to powders made of cornstarch or arrowroot. Lush and The Body Shop, for instance, both make them. Alternatively, here are some ultra-simple recipes if you'd like to try making your own.

Once you've mastered the basic recipe for body lotion, body oil, and dusting powders (opposite), you can adapt the blend of essential oils or base oils you use to suit your mood.

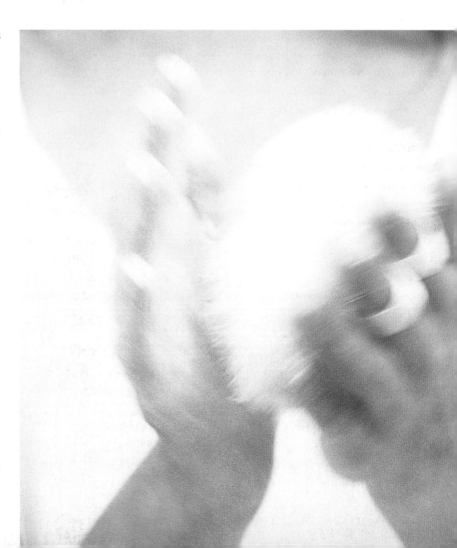

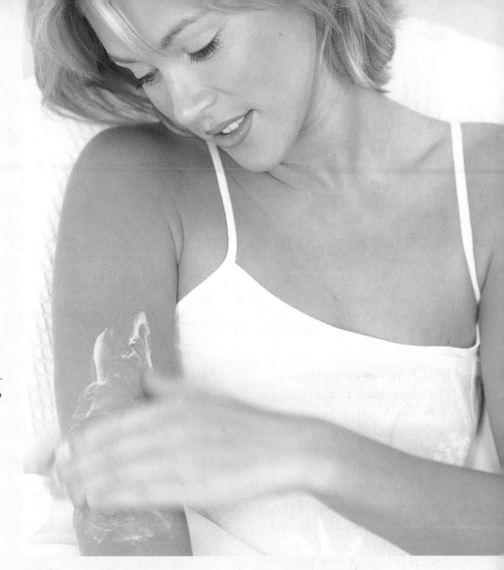

Rejuvenating body oil

This soothes and replenishes even the thirstiest, flakiest skin – and is perfect for just-got-back-from-vacation bodies.

½ cup (100 ml) glycerin

1 tsp wheatgerm oil

1½ tsp sweet almond oil

2 tsp jojoba oil

2 tsp sunflower oil

3 tbs distilled water

10 drops lemon juice

6 drops rose oil

6 drops neroli oil

3 drops chamomile oil

Beat the ingredients together in a ceramic bowl until everything is perfectly blended. Store in an airtight bottle with a spray top in a dark, cool place (or refrigerate), and always shake well before use. Use long, strong strokes to massage into skin.

Winter body oil

When skin is at its most parched, try this luxurious oil. Use after bathing, and anytime on chapped areas.

¼ cup (50 ml) avocado oil

2 tbs sweet almond oil

2 tbs apricot kernel oil

2 tbs olive oil

25 drops essential oil (use your favorites), for fragrance

Pour into a jar and shake until well blended. Bottle and store away from light.

Lavender dusting powder

⅓ cup (50 g) white kaolin clay

⅓ cup (50 g) arrowroot powder

⅓ cup (50 g) cornstarch

5 drops each lavender, clary sage, and mandarin essential oils

Combine the dry ingredients in a blender. Then add the essential oils and blend again. Decant the powder into a salt shaker for easy dusting onto the body; or pat it in a container and use a powderpuff.

Exotic dusting powder

Follow the instructions for Lavender Dusting Powder, but replace the essential oils with:

5 drops sandalwood oil

5 drops patchouli oil

2 drops frankincense oil

2 drops vetiver oil

Geranium body powder

1 cup (150 g) cornstarch

10 scented geranium leaves, washed and dried with a cloth

1-2 drops geranium essential oil

Pour the cornstarch into a jar and add the fresh leaves and the essential oil. Seal the lid, and shake. Shake the container once every day for 3-4 days, after which you can remove the leaves.

The powder can be poured into a clean, dry container – a flour shaker is ideal. Alternatively, apply it to the body using a large powder puff.

at-home
spa

There's no need to pay a fortune to escape to a spa. With a little preparation, you can leave reality behind and experience the benefits of a spa retreat, without even leaving home.

Most of us dream of spa getaways. But as with so many dreams, real life gets in the way. What is occasionally possible, with a little forward planning, is to turn off the world for an hour, a half-day, or even a day, to seize the opportunity to feel a little more pampered and beautiful.

Don't think of this time as selfish. Think of it as taking care of yourself, replenishing your reserves so you are better able to take care of everyone and everything in your busy life.

Setting aside time for yourself can enhance not only your appearance but also your overall wellbeing. "Simple, sensual acts such as touching and bathing can improve self-esteem, as well as reducing anxiety," says psychologist Dr. Cary Cooper.

Mix and match the treatments from this book according to the time available. Here's a suggested schedule for a half-day, which could easily be adapted to an evening.

- 9 a.m. Vegetable juice breakfast
- 9:15 a.m. Skin brushing
- 9:30 a.m. Head massage
- 9:45 a.m. Face mask
- 10 a.m. Reviving bath or invigorating shower
- 10:15 a.m. Yoga or stretching exercises
- 10:45 a.m. Foot massage and pedicure
- 11:30 a.m. Holistic manicure
- Midday. Organic lunch followed by your choice of herbal tea.

BE PREPARED

In order to maximize the pleasure of your at-home spa experience, make sure everything you need is ready in advance. Dashing to the store for last-minute things you've forgotten will seriously impact on your pleasure and relaxation.

- Plenty of purified or spring water to drink during your treatments.
- A pile of fluffy towels and a terrycloth bathrobe, if you have one.
- Scented candles or an aromatherapy

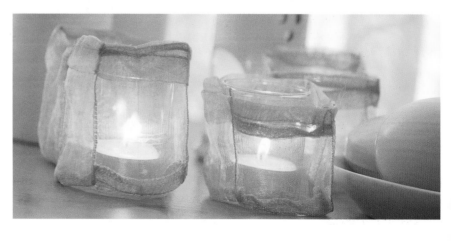

burner (for use with essential oils).

- Pumice stone and/or a foot file.
- Body brush, loofah, or washcloth.
- Organic fruit and vegetables for juicing and snacking.
- Essential oils.
- Any other ingredients for the treatments that you don't stock in your pantry or refrigerator.
- If you are going to treat yourself to a manicure or pedicure, you will need a hoof stick, orangewood sticks, nail polish remover, base coat, top coat, and the polish of your choice, plus toe dividers, if you want to use them.
- If you like to listen to music while pampering yourself, make a pile of all your favorite relaxing cassettes and CDs. Buy batteries for your CD/cassette player: it is extremely dangerous to have a stereo plugged into a socket if you are listening to music in the bathroom.

TOWELS GO ORGANIC

As explained on page 29, cotton is the most heavily sprayed crop on the planet; however, organic cotton towels are now available, although not, as yet, very widely. Next time you are replacing your towels, consider investing in the organic version – for your own pleasure and for the planet's sake. At the very least, go for unbleached towels. They feel as soft on the skin as conventional cotton towels, are just as absorbent, and come in a choice of back-to-nature, sense-soothing cream and off-white tones, rather than the rainbow shades of conventional towels.

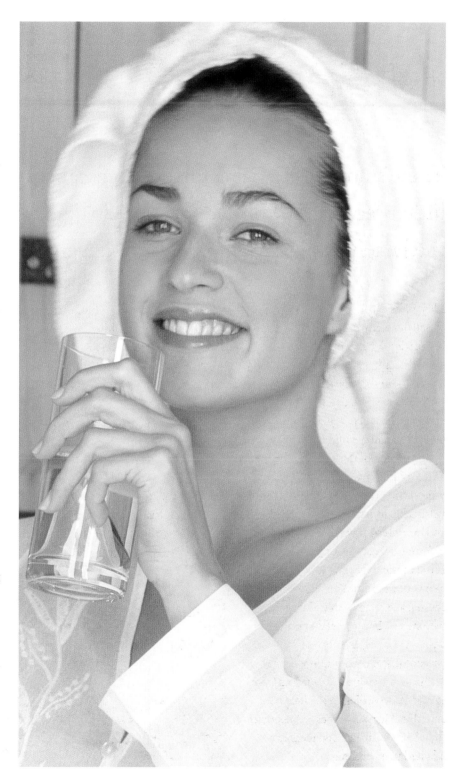

natural *deodorants*

To banish body odor we reach for an arsenal of pore-blocking ingredients that interfere with this natural body process. But natural alternatives will leave you smelling sweet.

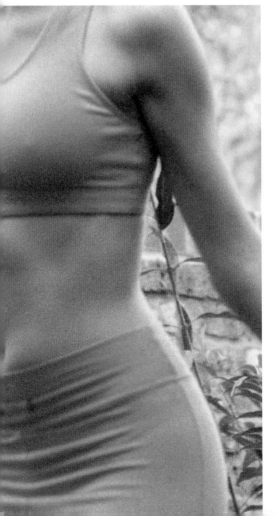

In a sanitized world, smelling of sweat has become unacceptable. Ironic, really, considering it is the pheromones (the musky sex hormones) in sweat that we seek to eliminate.

Our bodies have two types of sweat glands: eccrine and apocrine. The eccrine glands act as the body's thermostat, and their sweat has no smell. Odor comes from the apocrine glands (under the arms, around the nipples, and in the genital area). Made up mainly of water and salt, the sweat is fairly benign until it comes into contact with the skin's bacteria, which feed on sweat and break it down, causing body odor.

Pharmacies offer a huge selection of sweat-busters, but many are made up of myriad chemicals. Propylene glycol, for instance, is used in brake fluid and antifreeze and is linked in some studies to contact dermatitis, kidney damage, and liver abnormalities. Triclosan, a broad-spectrum antibacterial agent,

has been found in some instances to cause allergic contact dermatitis and, over the long term, to cause liver damage in animals. In addition, fears have been expressed that the widespread use of triclosan, used in hand washes and impregnated into some kitchen equipment, might encourage "superbug" bacteria.

Antiperspirants take sweat control one stage further, trying to stop it by blocking the pores with aluminum compounds: aluminum zirconium or aluminum chlorohydrate. These need to remain in the pores for a long time to work effectively, so they are easily absorbed into the bloodstream. According to a study published in the *Journal of Clinical Epidemiology*, "a statistically significant trend emerged between an increasing lifetime use of aluminum-containing antiperspirants and the estimated relative risk of Alzheimer's disease." So far, however, only one study has made this link.

"Rock" deodorants used for centuries in Asia are also based on aluminum salts. Unlike commercial antiperspirants, the deodorant (which is used by wetting a clear crystal stone and rubbing it on) does not stop perspiration, only odor. Whether these stones are 100 percent safe or not, however, is still a matter of contention in holistic health circles.

Naturopaths are also warning of another danger of antiperspirants: blocking underarm sweat can cause a buildup of toxins, and it has been suggested that heavy antiperspirant use could be contributing to the rising rate of breast cancer. Conventional medical researchers discount this, and it will be several years before studies weigh in, but it is worth remembering that sweat is the body's way to excrete toxins and waste products.

So, how can we stay sweet-smelling naturally? There are plenty of natural odor-busters in natural food stores, many of which avoid the ingredients listed above. Some are alcohol-based, and according to natural health guru Dr. Andrew Weil you could just rub alcohol under your arm, since it acts as an antibacterial agent. Check out those by Tom's of Maine, Weleda, Desert Essence, Dr. Hauschka, Aubrey Organics, Neal's Yard, Logona, and The Body Shop, among others. Origins, too, has formulated its No Offense deodorant without aluminum. You could also make your own: try a dusting of baking soda (a terrific deodorizer), arrowroot, or cornstarch.

Deodorant recipe

¼ cup (50 ml) vodka
2 tbs witch hazel
10 drops lavender oil
1 drop juniper oil
1 drop lemon oil

Combine all the ingredients in a sterilized pump-lid bottle, and shake before each use. This unisex blend works on both sexes. (Note: like most deodorants, it also stings if you use it after shaving!)

AEROSOL ALERT

Aerosol deodorants may be quick and easy to use, but each burst from the nozzle leaves you breathing in tiny droplets of what is in the can – together with the propellants, usually propane or butane. As a rule, they're not recyclable, either. So use pump-action sprays in glass bottles wherever practical.

Hair removal

You need to get only a whiff of hair-removing creams – which work by dissolving the hair – to know that they are packed with chemicals. Do you really want those on your skin? Shaving is the quickest and least messy way of hair removal. But if you want a technique that delivers longer-lasting results, try "sugaring," which is widely used in the Middle East. It can be tricky – and sticky – to perfect, but delivers smooth, stubble-free skin that can remain hair-free for up to 8 weeks.

To start with, try the following recipe, which is based on equal amounts of water and sugar:

1 tbs water
1 tbs granulated organic sugar

Mix the ingredients together in a metal pan over gentle heat. When the sugar has dissolved and the liquid is the consistency of honey, let it cool slightly until it is like toffee; when it reaches body temperature, apply it to the skin with a wooden spoon or a spatula. Place a strip of cotton over the top and press it onto your skin with your hands. Let it set thoroughly and pull the cotton off, remembering to pull against the direction in which the hair grows.

This recipe makes a very small quantity (for practicing!). As your technique improves, you can make bigger batches, remembering to keep the quantities equal. As an alternative, you can substitute lemon juice for the water.

If the skin is tender afterward, apply tea tree oil on a cotton pad to the area that has been depilated.

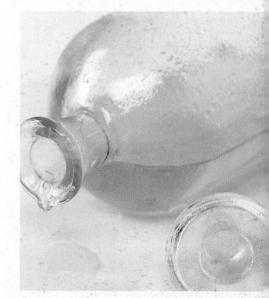

organic
fragrances

Women love perfume, but because fragrance manufacturers aren't obliged to list the precise contents of their products, organic beauties may wish to consider natural alternatives.

Perfume. It has been used it to beguile, seduce, and express individuality for centuries – dating back to well before the time of Cleopatra – but modern fragrance is a world away from the ancient perfumer's art.

NATURAL OR SYNTHETIC?

Most fragrances today are a combination of hundreds of different ingredients: some are natural elements, but most are synthetic. Some of those chemicals, for instance methylene chloride, may even be carcinogenic. Synthetics are used because they are far less expensive to produce. Fragrance industry "noses" also argue that synthetic ingredients do not vary, as natural elements can, differing subtly according to the soil they were grown on, the climate, and the speed with which they were processed.

A fragrance may contain as many as 200 different chemical ingredients, and because of the highly competitive nature of the business, it is impossible to tell what's in a fragrance – listing ingredients is tantamount to giving away a multimillion-dollar formula. Some consumer groups, however, are lobbying for labeling on fragrances, so that people with chemical sensitivities know what to avoid.

MAKE IT UP

Fragrance has become so much a part of our image that it is almost inconceivable to think of giving it up: a spritz to boost confidence, a dab for romance, a splash to cool down. It is up to you to decide your priorities and whether, instead of buying another bottle of perfume, you might like to have fun making your own.

Some natural food stores, meanwhile, carry all-natural fragrances from companies including Dr. Hauschka and the Australian brand, Natio (see *Directory* pages 122-124).

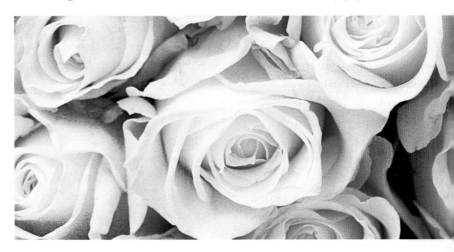

Carmelite water

This unisex cologne was first made by Carmelite monks in Paris in 1611.

1 generous handful angelica leaves

1 generous handful lemon balm leaves

1 tbsp lightly crushed coriander seeds

1 nutmeg, grated

2 tbsp cloves

3 pieces cinnamon stick, crushed

1¼ cups 80 proof (or higher) vodka

⅓ cup distilled water

Place all the spices and herbs in a wide-mouthed glass jar, then pour in the vodka. Seal and shake vigorously. Leave in a warm corner for a week to 10 days, shaking at least once a day. Strain through cheesecloth, then let the fragrant water drip through a coffee filter into a bottle. Dilute to the strength you want with more distilled water. Store away from light in a beautiful bottle.

Summer splash

Did you ever play in a greenhouse, rubbing your fingers on leaves and inhaling the mossy scents? This delicious summer scent combines the fragrance of geranium leaves with the tang of tomatoes.

4 tbsp fresh tomato leaves, chopped

2 tbsp scented geranium leaves, chopped

1 tsp fresh mint leaves

1 tbsp grated lemon rind

1 cup vodka or witch hazel

¼ teaspoon glycerin

Place the leaves and the grated lemon rind in a clean bottle then pour on the alcohol or witch hazel, together with the glycerin. Cover and let it sit in a cool, dark place for at least two weeks, before straining the liquid and discarding the solids. Pour into a sterilized spray bottle with a tight-fitting lid, and splash on. If you keep it cool, it's even more refreshing.

Solid perfume

This is a great way to carry perfume, because it's non-spill. Pour the mix, made in the same way as a lip balm, into a pillbox or a small pretty tin, and you can carry it in your handbag.

½ tbsp beeswax

4 tbsp almond oil

8 drops of essential oil

The following essential oils make great fragrance elements; play with them to create your own unique blends.

Tangerine	**Grapefruit**
Sandalwood	**Sweet orange**
Patchouli	**Geranium**
Vanilla	**Lemon**
Ylang-ylang	

In a small saucepan, gently heat the beeswax and oil until the wax is melted. Remove from the heat and stir in the essential oils; pour the mixture into a clean container. Let it cool, soften it with your fingers, and apply it to pulse points.

Note: most essential oils cannot be applied directly onto skin and must always be diluted with a carrier oil. Only lavender, tea tree, and peppermint can be used on their own – and you probably don't want to smell of the last two!

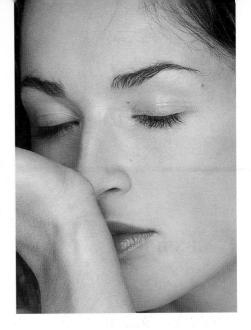

FRAGRANCE MEDITATION

The individual powers of essential oils are well-documented – citrus oils to invigorate, lavender for rebalancing, marjoram to relax – but behavioral psychologist Dr. Susan Schiffman, of Duke Univeristy Medical Center in North Carolina, believes it is possible to use any perfume to manage moods.

You need a back-supporting chair and a favorite scent. Sitting down, take three deep, languid breaths. Envision breathing relaxation in and tension out. In turn, stretch, tense, then relax your toes, legs, and abdomen. Make fists, flex your biceps, then relax. Shrug your shoulders. Scrunch your eyes and forehead, take a deep breath, and relax. Then bring the fragrance to your nose, inhale deeply – and try to maintain that sense of peace and quiet. Tell yourself that next time you smell the fragrance, the feeling will return.

Schiffman's subjects repeated the exercise once or twice daily: it took between one and 10 sessions before relaxation became a trigger response.

directory

Academy of Natural Living
132 Collins Avenue
Edge Hill
Cairns Qld 4870
Australia
Tel: 0061 7 4053 7786
academy.natural.living@iig.com.au

Aesop
71-79 Bouverie Street
Carlton
Melbourne 3053
Australia
Inquiries: 0061 3 9347 3422
Fax: 00 61 3 9347 3466
Website: www.aesop.net.au
Available in the U.S. through all Barneys New York
stores. For a full listing and detailed technical
information please refer to the website.

**Allergy Sensitivity and Environmental
Health Association**
PO Box 96
Margate Qld 4019
Australia
Tel: 0061 7 3284 8742
Fax: 0061 7 3284 8742
Website: www.asehaqld.org.au

Annemarie Börlind
c/o Simply Nature
Unit 7, Old Factory Buildings
Battenhurst Road
Stonegate
East Sussex TN5 7DU
UK
Mail order/inquiries: 00 44 1580 201687
Fax: 00 44 1580 201697

Aromantic
4 Heathneuk
Findhorn
IV36 3YY
UK
Mail order/inquiries: 00 44 1309 692000
Fax: 00 44 1309 691100
(organise courses in making your own beauty
products)

Aromatherapy Associates
68 Maltings Place
Bagleys Lane
Fulham
London SW6 2BY
UK
Mail order/inquiries: 00 44 20 7371 9878
Fax: 00 44 20 7371 9894
Website: www.aromatherapyassociates.com

Aubrey Organics (US)
4419 North Manhattan Avenue
Tampa, FL 33614
Mail order/inquiries: 1 800 282 7394
Fax: 1 813 876 8166
Website: www.aubrey-organics.com

**Australasian College of Natural
Therapies**
57 Fouveaux Street
Surry Hills NSW 2010
Australia
Tel: 0061 2 9218 8850
Fax: 0061 2 9281 4411
info@acnt.edu.au

Australian Homeopathic Association
PO Box 396
Drummoyne NSW 2047
Australia
Tel: 0061 2 9719 2793
Tas: 0061 3 6267 9877
WA: 0061 8 929 4258
SA: 0061 8 8388 9145
Qld: 0061 7 3371 7245
Vic: 0061 3 5979 3203
Fax: 0061 2 9719 2763
Website: www.aushom.asn.au

Australian Institute of Holistic Medicine
PO Box 3079
Jandakot WA 6164
Tel: 0061 8 9417 3553
Fax: 0061 8 9417 1881
info@aihm.wa.edu.au
Website: www.aihm.wa.edu.au

Aveda
AVD Cosmetics
7 Munton Road, London SE17 1PR
UK
Mail order/inquiries: 00 44 20 7410 1600
Fax: 00 44 20 7410 1899
Website: www.aveda.com

Bare Escentuals (US)
425 Bush Street
3rd Floor
San Francisco, CA 94108
Mail order/inquiries: 1 800 227 3990
Fax: 001 415 288 3501
Website: www.bareescentuals.com

Beauty and the Bees
60 Cambridge Road
Bellerive Tas 7018
Australia
bebeauty@netspace.net.au
Website: www.beebeauty.com

Bioforce (UK) Limited
2 Brewster Place
Irvine
Ayrshire KA11 5DD
UK
Mail order/inquiries: 00 44 1294 277 344
Fax: 00 44 1294 277 922
www.bioforce.co.uk

British Union of Anti-Vivisection (BUAV)
16a Crane Grove
London N7 8NN
UK
Inquiries: 00 44 20 7700 4888
Fax: 00 44 20 7700 0252
Website: www.buav.org

Burt's Bees
PO Box 13489
Durham, NC 27709
Mail order/inquiries: 1 800 849 7112
Fax: 1 800 429 7487
Website: www.burtsbees.com

Cariad
Rivernook Farm
Sunnyside
Walton on Thames
Surrey KT12 2ET
UK
Mail order/inquiries: 00 44 1932 269 921
Fax: 00 44 1932 253 220
Website: www.cariad.co.uk

Caudalie
9 Villa Aublet
75017 Paris
France
Mail order/inquiries:
Fax: 00331 44 29 24 25
Website: www.caudalie.com

Clarins
Clarins UK Limited
10 Cavendish Place
London W1G 9DN
UK
Mail order/inquiries: 00 44 20 7307 6700
Fax: 00 44 20 7307 6701
Website: www.clarins.co.uk

Colorings
The Body Shop
Watersmead
Littlehampton
West Sussex BN17 6LS
UK
Inquiries: 00 44 1903 731500
Fax: 00 44 1903 844383
Website: www.the-body-shop.com

Comfort & Joy
Baytree Cottage
Eastleach
Nr Cirencester
Gloucestershire GL7 3NL
UK
Mail order/inquiries & Fax: 00 44 1367 850278

Daniel Field
8-12 Broadwick Street
London W1V 1FH
UK
Mail order/inquiries: 00 44 20 7437 1490
or 00 44 20 7439 8223 (salon)
Fax: 00 44 20 7287 4954

Decléor
59a Connaught Street
London W2 2BB
UK
Mail order/inquiries: 00 44 20 7402 9474
Fax: 00 44 20 7262 1886
Website: www.decleor–co.uk

Desert Essence
Crest House
102-104 Church Road
Teddington
Middlesex TW11 8PY
UK
Mail order/inquiries: 00 44 800 146 215
Fax: 00 44 20 8614 1422
Website: www.country-life.com

Dr. Hauschka
Unit 19/20 Stockwood Business Park
Stockwood
Nr. Redditch
Worcestershire B96 6SX
UK
Mail order/inquiries: 00 44 1527 832863
Fax: 00 44 1386 792623
Website: www.drhauschka.co.uk

Ecover
c/o Beasley & Christopher
21 Castle Street
Brighton BN1 2HD
UK
Mail order/inquiries: 00 44 1273 206997
Fax: 00 44 1273 206973
Website: www.ecover.com

Elemis
The Lodge
92 Uxbridge Road
Harrow Weald
Middlesex HA3 6BZ
UK
Mail order/inquiries: 00 44 20 8954 8033
Fax: 00 44 20 8909 5030
Website: www.elemis.com

E'SPA
21 East Street
Farnham
Surrey GU9 7SD
UK
Mail order/inquiries: 00 44 1252 741600
Fax: 00 44 1252 742810

Eve Lom
2 Spanish Place
London W1U 3HU
UK
Mail order/inquiries: 00 44 20 8661 7991

Everest Hill Aromas
E'SPA House
Hill House
Kingston Hill
Surrey KT2 7LB
UK
Mail order/inquiries: 00 44 20 8546 7665
Email: EHA@hillheights.demon.co.uk

Farmacia
169 Drury Lane
Covent Garden
London WC2B 5QA
UK
Mail order/inquiries: 00 44 20 7404 8808
Website: www.farmacia123.com

Gowings
Level 8
45 Market Street
Sydney NSW 2000
Australia
Tel: 0061 1800 803 304
Fax: 0061 2 9261 3020
worldstore@gowings com.au
Website: www.gowings.com.au

The Green People Company
Brighton Road
Handcross
West Sussex RH17 6BZ
UK
Mail order/inquiries: 00 44 1444 401444
Fax: 00 44 1444 401011
Website: www.greenpeople.co.uk

The Health Emporium
263 Bondi Road
Bondi NSW 2026
Australia
Tel: 0061 2 9365 6008
Fax: 0061 2 9300 9330

Herb Research Foundation
1007 Pearl Street
Suite 200
Boulder, CO 80302
Mail order/inquiries: 1 303 449 2265
Fax: 1 303 449 7849
Website: www.herbs.org

Jane Iredale
Iredale Mineral Cosmetics
121 Cambridge Road
Wimpole
Near Royston
Hertfordshire SG8 5QB
UK
Mail order/inquiries: 00 44 800 328 2467
Fax: 00 44 1223 208507
Website: www.janeiredale.com

Jurlique
Naturopathic Health & Beauty Co
Willowtree Marina
West Quay Drive
Yeading
Middlesex UB4 9TB
UK
Mail order/inquiries: 00 44 20 8841 6644
Fax: 00 44 20 8841 7557
Website: www.jurlique.com.au
(product prices for Australia only)

Just Pure
PO Box 1113
Lechbruck Am See
Germany
Mail order/inquiries: 0049 836 7789
Fax: 0049 836 7808
Website: www.justpure.com

Lavera
Laverana GmbH
Am Weingarten 4
D - 30974 Wennigsen
Germany
Telefon: 0049 5103 93910
Telefax: 0049 5103 939139
Mail order/inquiries:
(c/o Farmacia, UK) 00 44 20 7404 8808

Living Nature
The Old Milkhouse
Manor Farm
Rockbourne
Hampshire SP6 3NP
IK
Mail order/inquiries: 00 44 1725 518072
Fax: 00 44 1725 518073
Website: www.livingnature.com
Email: livnature@aol.com

Liz Earle
PO Box 50
Ryde
Isle of Wight PO33 2YD
UK
Mail order/inquiries: 00 44 1983 813913
Fax: 00 44 1983 812333
Website: www.lizearle.com

Logona
Unit 3B, Beck's Green Business Park
Beck's Green Lane
Ilketshall St. Andrew
Beccles
Suffolk NR34 8NB
UK
Mail order/inquiries: 00 44 1986 781782
Fax: 00 44 1449 780 297
Website: www.logona.co.uk

Lush
29 High Street
Poole
Dorset BH15 1AB
UK
Mail order/inquiries: 00 44 1202 668545
Fax: 00 44 1202 661832
Website: www.lush.co.uk

Moor Mud
Austrian Moor Products
Moor House
7 Swift Close
East Sussex TN22 5PY
UK
Inquiries: 00 44 1825 765678

Nad's
31 Maryon Mews
London NW3 2PU
UK
Mail order/inquiries: 00 44 870 789 8010
Fax: 00 44 20 7813 7130

Natural Care College and Clinic
79 Lithgow Street
St Leonards NSW 2065
Australia
Tel: 0061 2 9438 3333
Fax: 0061 2 9436 0503

Natura Health 2000
Guthrey Centre
Cashel Street
City Mall
Christchurch
New Zealand
Tel: 0061 4 379 0451
Fax: 0061 4 329 9400

Natio
6 Paterson Street
Abbotsford
Melbourne Victoria 3067
Australia
Mail order/inquiries: 00613 9415 9911
Fax: 0061 3 9415 9922
Website: www.natio.com.au

Neal's Yard Remedies
26-34 Ingate Place
London SW8 3NS
UK
Inquiries: 00 44 20 7627 1949
Mail order: 00 44 161 831 7875
Fax: 020 7498 2505
Website: www.nealsyardremedies.com

Neem Organics
PO Box 307
Berry NSW 2535
Australia
Tel: 0061 2 4464 2674
Fax: 0061 2 4464 2648
sales@neem.com.au
www.neem.com.au

Neways International UK Limited
Harvard Way
Huntingdon
Cambridgeshire PE28 0NN
UK
Distributor inquiries: 00 44 1480 861764
Fax: 00 44 1480 861771
Website: www.neways.com

NHR Organic Oils
10 Bamborough Gardens
London W12 8QN
UK
Mail order/inquiries: 00 44 800 074 7744
Fax: 00 44 845 310 8068
Website: www.nhr.kz

Origins
73 Grosvenor Street
London W1X 0BH
UK
Mail order/inquiries: 00 44 800 731 4039
Fax: 00 44 20 7409 6827
Website: www.origins.com

Patagonia
397 Kent Street
Sydney NSW 2000
Australia
Tel: 0061 2 9264 2500/1800 066 625
Fax: 0061 2 9264 2505
sydney@patagonia.com.au

Phytothérathie/Phytologie
6 Bankside Buildings
9 Risborough Street
London SE1 0HF
UK
Mail order/inquiries: 00 44 20 7620 1771
Fax: 00 44 20 7620 1593

REN
40 Liverpool Street
London EC2M 7QN
UK
Mail order/inquiries: 00 44 20 7618 5353
Website: www.ren.ltd.uk

Shu Uemura
Unit 19
49 Atalanta Street
London SW6 6TU
UK
Mail order/inquiries: 00 44 20 7379 6627
Fax: 00 44 20 7386 0997
Website: www.shu-uemura.co.jp

Spectrum Oils (Essential Max)
Clear Spring
19a Acton Park Estate
London W3 7QE
UK
Mail order/inquiries: 00 44 20 8746 0152
Fax: 00 44 20 8811 8893
Website: www.clearspring.co.uk

The Soil Association
40-56 Victoria Street
Bristol BS1 6BY
UK
Inquiries: 00 44 117 929 0661
Fax: 00 44 117 925 2504
Website: www.soilassociation.org

Tom's of Maine
PO Box 710
Kennebunk, ME 04043
Mail order/inquiries: 1 800 775 2388
or 1 207 985 2944
Fax: 1 207 985 2196
Website: www.tomsofmaine.com

Trevarno Organic Skincare
Trevarno Estate and Gardens
Helston
Cornwall TR13 0RU
UK
Tel: 00 44 1326 574274
Fax: 00 44 1326 574282

Tweezerman
c/o Luxe
3-5 Barrett Street
London W1U 1AY
UK
Mail order: 00 44 20 7629 1234 (Selfridges)

Udo's Choice
Savant Distribution Ltd.
15 Iveson Approach
Ireland Wood
Leeds LS16 6LJ
UK
Mail order/inquiries: 00 44 113 230 1993
Fax: 00 44 113 230 1915
Website: www.savant-health.com

Urtekram
c/o Marigold
102 Camley Street
London NW1 0PF
UK
Mail order/inquiries: 00 44 20 7388 4515
Fax: 00 44 20 7388 4516

Weleda
Heanor Road
Ilkeston
Derbyshire DE7 8DR
UK
Mail order/inquiries: 00 44 115 944 8200
Fax: 00 44 115 944 8210
Website: www.weleda.co.uk

Woodspirits
Unit 42, New Lydenburg Industrial Estate
New Lydenburg Street
London SE7 8NE
UK
Tel: 00 44 208293 4949
Fax: 00 44 208293 4949

Yin Yang
Unit C1
New Yatt Centre
Witney
Oxfordshire OX8 6TJ
UK
Mail order/inquiries: 00 44 1993 868 912
Fax: 00 44 1993 868 628
Website: www.yinyang.co.uk

FURTHER READING
The Safe Shopper's Bible: A Consumer,s Guide to
Nontoxic Household Products, Cosmetics and
Food by David Steinman and Samuel S. Epstein,
M.D. (IDG Books Worldwide, $14.95)

What's In Your Cosmetics? By Aubrey Hampton
(Organica Press, $11)

The Handmade Soap Book by Melinda Coss (New
Holland, $22.95)

A Consumers Dictionary of Cosmetic Ingredients
by Ruth Winter (Three Rivers Press, $16)

glossary

These are some of the ingredients you will find on labels, together with some of the widely-used terms. The ingredients are listed in Latin, with their English translation in brackets.

Aesculus hippocastanum (horse chestnut) good for circulation, has an astringent action

Alcohol (ethanol) used as a highly effective preservative. However, ethanol can increase the skin's permeability and may enhance absorption of ingredients, including chemicals

Allantoin derived from comfrey root, this is healing and soothing to irritated skin

Aloe barbadensis (aloe vera) soothing, cooling, with anti-irritant and healing powers

Ananas sativus (pineapple extract) containing mild fruit acids to cleanse and exfoliate the skin

Apple cider vinegar helps balance the natural acidity of skin and hair, and remove dead skin cells

Aqua (water) usually the No. 1 item in manufactured cosmetics

Ascorbic acid (vitamin C) a natural preservative, antioxidant and skin pH balancer

Butyrospermum parkii (shea butter) highly compatible with skin, this is an excellent moisturizer with skin-healing properties

Calcium carbonate (chalk) a gentle abrasive

Calendula officinalis (pot marigold) soothing and healing to irritated, inflamed or delicate skin, with some antiseptic properties

Cannabis sativa (hemp seed oil) rich in fatty acids and minerals that have skin and hair benefits

Cetearyl alcohol may be naturally- or chemically-derived, this is used as an emollients, emulsifier and/or thickener

Cetyl alcohol see cetearyl alcohol

Chamaemelum recutita (chamomile extract) soothing

Cinnamonum zeylanicum (cinnamon oil) antimicrobial, antiseptic

Citric acid pH modifier

Citrus grandis (grapefruit seed extract) antiseptic and preservative

Citrus paradisi (grapefruit essential oil) astringent, antiseptic, rich in vitamin C

Citrus sinensis (orange essential oil) antiseptic, refreshing

Cocos nucifera (coconut oil) an excellent emollient

Elaeis guineensis (palm kernel oil) emollient and skin-lubricant

Foeniculum vulgare (fennel oil) antiseptic, antimicrobial and anti-inflammatory

Glycerin derived from plants, this is a humectant (attracting water to the skin), emollient, emulsifier and solvent

Gnaphalium leontopodium (Edelweiss extract) high in antioxidants, helps protect against UV radiation

Hamamelis virginiana (witch hazel) astringent, pore-tightening

Hedera helix (ivy) used for its toning powers in anti-cellulite potions

Helianthus annuus (sunflower oil) richly lubricating and emollient

Humulus lupulus (hops) a gentle skin toner

Lavandula angustifolia (lavender essential oil) soothing, healing, balancing and calming, as well as antiseptic; good for sensitive and delicate skin

Melaleuca alternifolia (tea tree essential oil) powerful antiseptic, antifungal, antiviral; helps keep skin/scalp infection-free

Mentha piperita (peppermint oil) good for combating bad breath

Montmorillonite (pink clay) cleansing, absorbent, to help draw out impurities

Oenothera biennis (evening primrose oil) a rich source of omega-3 and omega-6 fatty acids, good for dry skin conditions

Olea europaea (olive oil) emollient and lubricant, it also strengthens the hair shaft

Pelargonium graveolens (geranium essential oil) useful for balancing all skin conditions

Persea gratissima (avocado oil) rich in vitamins D, E and beta-carotene, emollient, hydrating, moisturizing and nourishing

Prunus armeniaca (apricot seed oil) lubricating and nourishing

Rose spp. (extract of damask, centifolia, and/or gallica roses) helps to maintain the skin's natural moisture balance, it's particularly good for inflamed, itchy or mature skins

Rosemarinus officinalis (rosemary essential oil) refreshing, invigorating, stimulating for skin; good for tackling scalp problems

Salvia officinalis (sage) astringent and antiseptic

Santalum alba (sandalwood essential oil) good for all skintypes, especially mature, dry and dehydrated skins

Sodium hydroxide (caustic soda) common ingredient in soap

Triticum vulgare (wheatgerm oil) rich in vitamin E and wonderful for dry skin

Unicaria tomentosa (cat's claw) stimulates the skin's natural immune system and is useful for sensitive skin

Vitis vinifera (grapeseed extract) mild fruit acids, to help exfoliate and cleanse skin

Titanium dioxide a physical UV filter, which bounces, the sun's rays off skin

Zinc oxide a physical UV filter

index

thanks...

Dorling Kindersley would like to thank the following companies for the kind loan of their natural products:

Aveda, AVD Cosmetics, 7 Munton Road, London SE17 1PR, UK Tel: 00 44 20 7410 1600

Damask, Unit 7, Sullivan Enterprise Centre, Sullivan Road, London SW6, UK Tel: 00 44 20 77313470

David Mellor, 4 Sloane Square, London SW1, UK Tel: 00 44 20 7730 4259

Dr. Hauschka, Unit 19/20 Stockwood Business Park, Stockwood, Worcestershire, B96 6SX, UK Tel: 00 44 1527 832863

Farmacia, 169 Drury Lane, Covent Garden, London WC2B 5QA, UK Tel: 00 44 20 7404 8808

Jurlique, Naturopathic Health & Beauty Co, Willowtree Marina, West Quay Drive, Yeading, Middlesex UB4 9TB, UK Tel: 00 44 20 8841 6644

Neal's Yard, 26-34 Ingate Place, Battersea, London SW8 3NS, UK Tel: 00 44 20 7627 1949

Origins, 73 Grosvenor Street, London W1X OBH, UK Tel: 00 44 800 731 4039

Voodoo Blue, Unit 10, Brentford Business Park, Commerce Road, Brentford, Middlesex, TW8 8LG, UK Tel: 00 44 20 8560 7050

Woodspirits, Unit 42, New Lydenburg Industrial Estate, New Lydenburg Street, London SE6 8NE, UK Tel: 00 44 20 8293 4949

The publisher would also like to thank the following people for the use of their homes as locations: John Davis; Gill Dickinson; Mary-Clare Jerram and Jimmy and Denny Wade.

The author would like to thank Liz Hancock, Sally Argyle, Renée Elliot, Lynda Brown, and above all Craig Sams.